20TH ANNIVERSARY EDITION

Author's Forward

Recently, a friend in the health and fitness industry was visiting and noticed the author's copy of my book, Diet Evolution.

She picked it up, thumbing through it and said, *"CJ, when did you write this book?"*

"Oh, about 20 years ago", I replied.

"This is amazing, you were talking Keto, long before we were using the term Keto to describe a diet. Maybe you should re-release this book", she said.

She was so enthusiastic, I decided to re-read my book and thought about why it did not get the traction that it could have. And then I recalled how a few events led to a disruption in its marketing and, without those opportunities, broad market publicity for the book was lost.

It was around September 2000 and I was to appear on a popular daytime talk show, ABC's *The View*, to discuss my book. Star Jones, a cohost who wanted to lose some weight, said during a previous show that she loved bacon, a food that was seriously frowned upon during the low-fat, high-carbohydrate diet years which was most popular at the time. I faxed the *The View*'s production office in New York and told them, on my diet, Star could eat bacon and still lose weight. They booked me to appear on the show about a week later. I was ecstatic.

Diet Evolution would be seen on *The View* by millions of viewers, and not only generate an increase in sales, but create a cascade of opportunities to help promote the book and this healthy *"Eat Fat, Get Fit"* way of life, something we now call KETO.

As it turned out, things change rapidly in daytime talk television, and *The View* got some great new ratings after my booking, and my slot was rebooked for a well-known celebrity. Of course, you can't blame them for doing what they think is best for the show. My agent told me *"they usually re-book guests that get bumped"* but unfortunately that was not the case for me. I would have loved to meet all the ladies in person to hear what they thought of the diet -- and my naked cover.

And so, with my friends bug in my ear, and renewed energy and belief in the relevance of the original message of this book, I decided to release a 20th anniversary e-book edition of *Diet Evolution*, dedicated to my father, Charles J Hunt Jr, who once told me ...*"Finding the right time for everything makes all the difference."*

My hope is that t*his is the right tim*e for Diet Evolution *to help you* achieve the health and life you deserve.

September 17, 2020
Charles "CJ" Hunt

CHARLES HUNT'S DIET EVOLUTION, 20TH ANNIVERSARY EDITION

Eat Fat and Get Fit!

Charles J Hunt

Hunt Thompson Media

The information contained in this book is from the Authors experiences and is not designed to replace the advice or care of your personal health care professional. - If you are taking a prescription medication, consult your health care professional as any dietary changes, good or bad, will affect the metabolism of your medication. The Author does not directly or indirectly dispense medical advice or prescribe the use of this diet and fitness program as a form of treatment.

Although this book, personal coaching and Diet Evolution seminars are based in using food as the foundation of any health improvement program, and they present what the Author believes to be the most advanced dietary understanding available at this time, the Publishers and Author expressly disclaim responsibility for any adverse effects arising from the use this diet and fitness program, or nutritional supplements, without the supervision of your health care professional - which we do advise.

Original paperback Library of Congress Catalog Card Number 99-90155
Hunt, Charles.
Charles Hunt's Diet Evolution (tm) "Eat Fat and Get Fit!"
ISBN: 0-9630377-1-4 Original Paperback
ISBN: 978-0-9630377-6-3 Ebook - Adobe PDF
ISBN: 978-0-9630377-5-6 Ebook - Kindle
ISBN: 978-0-9630377-9-4 Paperback - Kindle
1. Weight Loss 2. Nutrition
Cover Design & Book Layout: Steve Minard (c)1999 Charles Hunt
Diet Evolution Pyramid: Steve Minard (c)1999 Charles Hunt
Printed in USA

CONTENTS

20th Anniversary Edition
Title Page
Copyright
Part One 1
Chapter One 2
Chapter Two 11
Chapter Three 18
Chapter Four 28
Chapter Five 35
Part Two: A New you 38
Chapter Six 39
Chapter Seven 41
Chapter Eight 42
Chapter Nine 44
Chapter Ten 45
Chapter Eleven 47
Chapter Twelve 49
Chapter Thirteen 51
Part Three: Fitness 57
Chapter Fourteen 58

Chapter Fifteen	59
Chapter Sixteen	64
Chapter Seventeen	65
Chapter Eighteen	68
Chapter Nineteen	71
Chapter Twenty	79
Chapter Twenty-One	80
Part Four: Recipes	83
Beef	86
Beef, Ground	89
Veal	92
Lamb	95
Pork	98
Sausage	101
Baked Chicken	105
Crock Pot Chicken	108
Grilled and Broiled Chicken	112
Game Birds	115
Wild Game	117
Organ Meats	125
Fish	129
Shellfish	143
Shrimp	148
Lobster	154
Eggs	156
Vegetables	160
Meat Soups	173
Chicken Soups	175

Fish Soups	178
Vegetable Soups	180
Salads	185
Salad Dressings	191
Condiments	195
Chutneys	199
Stocks, Sauces & Gravies	203
Marinades	206
Rendering Fats	207
Dried Meats	208
Dry Rubs	211
Chili Powder	213
Hot Beverages	215
Cold Beverages	218
Nut Milks	220
Special Occasions	222
Fruits	226
Frozen Desserts	230
Dessert Sauces	233
Candy and Confections	234
Bread, pancakes, muffins, and cookies	236
Stuffing	239
About The Author	241
Resources	243
Books By This Author	245

PART ONE

Charles Hunt's Diet Evolution

1 HeartQuake
2 The Evolution of Diet
3 Death by Pyramid
4 Twilight of The Zone
5 Diet Evolution vs. The Popular Diets

CHAPTER ONE

Heartquake - My Story

Almost dying was the best thing that ever happened to me. I know this may sound a little weird to you, but it was. Don't worry, this is not a book about searching for your spirituality, and I didn't "see the light", or meet my grandmother and he dog as I crossed over to the other side. It wasn't like that at all. What did happen to me started a journey into the roots of health and fitness that not only saved but also vastly improved my life-and it can do the same for you.

On Memorial Day in 1978, my friend Stan wanted to jog with me at the local high school running track, not in the lush, green hillsides as was my custom. There is almost nothing I hated more than running in circles around a hot, dry and dusty track. *"OK just this once"* I said.

As we started, I ignored the fact that my breathing seemed unusually labored and heavy. We continued for a lap and a half, and I still wasn't shaking it off. I just wasn't feeling my normal 24-year-old "sparky" self. Something was "out of whack". I just thought I was a little tired, when, without warning, I felt extremely dizzy.

Realizing I was blacking out, I quickly turned towards the

grassy infield so I wouldn't get hurt on the track's rough gravel surface. My body, completely limp, hit the grass with a thud.

The next thing I remember feeling was my throat hurt. *"Better do something about that when I wake up,"* I thought. The pain grew incredibly fast, and soon I couldn't breathe. I thought that I'd swallowed a pencil or something similar and I had to pull it out quick! I tried to move to pull it out but nothing happened; I couldn't feel the rest of my body at all. By then I couldn't breathe and started crying as I panicked. A moment later, I felt something pulled from my throat and air rushed back into my lungs. It was an esophageal airway the paramedics had put down my throat while resuscitating me and applying electric shock to re-start my heart.

As feeling slowly returned to my limbs, I heard the muffled voice of my friend Stan calling out from somewhere in the distance among other voices saying that I "*had a heart attack or something*".

I felt my body being lifted, and the sounds closed around me, as I was moved into the ambulance. Voices started filtering in louder, a siren shrieked above me, and the paramedics started testing my level of consciousness asking me for my name, address and phone number to deter-mine the possibility of brain damage since I had been with-out oxygen for at least 4 minutes, and under CPR with little oxygen for about another ten minutes.

When we rolled into the emergency entrance of UCLA Medical Center, they said that they thought I was lucky. They didn't think I had any brain damage. I asked them how they could know, since they hadn't known me before!

There was too much happening too fast that my cut-up like nothing's wrong response kicked in, but I was getting scared. It was worse for me because there was no real warning. My heart had just stopped cold.

Over the next ten days, in intensive care, I learned what the doctor's thought had happened. I was to be put on drugs for the rest of my life, in an attempt to prevent this from happening again.

I was too stubborn to just give up and live on drugs, so I made some very scary choices, and I'm really glad I did. I'm glad for me, and I'm glad for you too because I'm here to share with you what saved my life. I learned what I needed to do to maximize my own genetic potential for health. In doing that, I also became leaner and stronger than I'd ever been. You can do it too.

This was not the first experience, but probably the most dramatic, in a really discouraging history of health problems to hit me over the years-from extreme low blood sugar to 42 lbs. of excess fat.

It may have taken me many years from that very scary day to solve my own health problems, but it didn't take me long to find out that these problems weren't just mine -they effect at least 75% of all of us.

Ultimately, it took me twenty years to figure out what we all need to do to avoid many very serious health problems, and stay remarkably lean, healthy and young-maximizing our total physical, mental and emotional potential for as long as possible. I call it the *DIET EVOLUTION.*

Just so we're clear on the matter, I'm not a doctor, *(I haven't even played one on TV - not yet anyway)*, or a registered dietitian, biochemist, or exercise physiologist. I'm a "regular guy", who just happens to be an investigative reporter with a somewhat dramatic, but extremely motivating health history. It sent me looking for new answers, and new questions. More importantly, when it comes to helping you to reach the best health and the leanest body you could ever have, I've got the experience to get you there. I'm a reporter who's actually "walked the walk" for twenty years now, religiously trying almost every nutritionally based lead I could dig up in the pursuit of health and wellness.

Like most of you, I've tried everything, from vegetarianism to fasting. Also, like most of you, I've often been overwhelmed by the non-stop media onslaught of contradictory, and oftentimes inaccurate health and nutrition information. Ineffective diet books, grossly excessive fitness regimes, rip-off supplement programs and short sighted, quick fixes are avail-able everywhere. It can be impossible to know what works and what doesn't. People can actually do themselves more harm than good. In fact, at one point in my broad-cast journalism career, in an effort to get lean, a combination of books led me to believe that power walking two hours a day like Oprah, and a Vegan raw food diet *(no meat, fish, eggs, dairy or cooked food)*, would do the trick.

It did, in a way. I got lean, really lean. But I also became listless, cranky, dispirited and completely worn out. Not what I'd call particularly healthy *(but if listless, cranky and worn out turns you on, I've got an old wheatgrass juicer you can have).*

Realistically, it's impossible for most of you to have the time to research all of the possibilities, and make effective, lifetime choices. That's one of the big reasons I've written this book for you and made it incredibly easy to follow. Think of me as your personal coach, simplifying the confusing mountains of research and "techno-babble", guiding you beyond the bookshelves filled with over-hyped, and overweight diet gurus. If you stopped and thought about it, if they don't at least look good following their own advice, you probably don't really want to go there *(by the way, that's me naked on the cover).*

I know what I have to share is valuable because I have a past of "down to earth", "in the trenches", real life experience. I'm not just another PhD. theorist interested in postulating assumptions, or proof gained from a limited population in a petri dish environment. Or quoting one short decade of questionable studies as the absolute truth. I'm only interested in getting to the heart of our national diet and fitness failure and finding out what actually works for most of us. As time goes on, if some of my current information can be upgraded, great! Besides, if I was one of the "hot-diets" of the month, I wouldn't have anything new to share.

As you read on, you'll see that my program will change your life forever.

Wake Up!

My personal wake-up call started at age 11, when an emergency appendectomy pulled me out of Boy Scout camp and left me with a large abdominal scar. *"The worst case in over thirty years"* they said.

By fourteen I started getting chubby, and suffering from what turned out to be acute hypoglycemia (low blood sugar) and all the frightening things that go with it. All because I loved that cinnamon toast every morning or Cheerios with enough sugar to hear it scrape through the milk from the bottom of the bowl. At that age who didn't go *"coo-Coo for Coco Puff's"*, or stick their ear into the bowl to listen for that famous *"Snap, Crackle, Pop!"*

But what we didn't know then, and still aren't "getting" now, is that about 75% of us are predisposed to blood sugar problems, eventually making us fat, sick and devitalized. Unfortunately, our moms didn't know any better either.

By seventeen, this diagnosis was confirmed when I was rushed from my high school to the hospital, after passing out during lunch break, but only after being accused of being on drugs by the Vice-principal who yelled nastily *"What are you on boy?!"* (the administration was *"Oh, so sorry"* after the blood tests came in).

At age twenty-one, my weight topped out at *230-pounds*. I had increased physical and emotional fragility, and rigorously tried every diet program I could find to feel and look better.

At the age of twenty-four I dropped dead from a cardiac arrest.

I spent the next ten days at the 4th Floor Cardiac Care Unit at UCLA Medical Center in Los Angeles and was eventually released with the following "to do" list:

1) Don't get your heart rate up over 120 beats per minute.

2) Don't walk upstairs.

3) Always be with someone who knows CPR. *(right!)*

4) Give up all sports.

5) Take beta-blocking (depressant) drugs four times a day for the rest of your life.

And, last but not least:

6) Maybe you'll survive sex *(I'm not joking).*

I mean, geez ... I was so shy as it was, sex was almost a non-issue, but now? In fact, the first time I ventured into love-making territory after this, I scared the hell out of my girlfriend. Just at our peak, I remembered the warning, grabbed my throat to find my pulse, looked at my wrist-watch, and started counting... *(Aaarrrghh!).*

Even though I was lucky enough to be jogging in the right place at the right time that Memorial Day in 1978, and I was grateful that I was kept alive by a passing anesthesiologist, until I was brought back to life by local paramedics, the future was looking very bleak.

> *When I insisted on exercising, the doctors at UCLA said I had a 50% chance of dying if I did, and they flatly refused to allow me into a medically supervised fitness group.*

So finally, in frustration, I ended up having my mother follow me in her car everyday so I could run, with some rescue close by. We both hoped that if I made it passed the first few minutes, I'd be OK.

It didn't take long for a life of medically-prescribed depressant drugs (those messed me up big time), little activity, and constant drop-dead-at-any-moment fear to get old. Believe it or not, they actually kicked me out of my active medical follow-up, because I wasn't willing to just sit around, slowly wasting away, doing nothing. I guess I'm just too naturally pro-active for some.

So, I decided that, for me, "quality of life" was more important than the vague hope of increased quantity. If this was all the medical world could offer, I had better figure out something for myself.

First, I weaned myself off prescription drugs and began a twenty-year process of research, experimentation and discovery.

Much of those twenty years was spent developing into an investigative news reporter. From that perspective, I had the unique opportunity to discover what looked to me like years and years of misinformation on health, nutrition and fitness hyped by the media. I had both the time and access to sort through mountains of international research and daily news releases. No matter what these various reports claimed, I kept coming across an equation that didn't add up, and still doesn't:

1 Based on all of the commonly accepted findings about diet and health,

+

2 The huge growth of health-consciousness of the American public.

= **3** We as a nation should be getting leaner and healthier.

But we're not.

The truth is, obesity and disease are on the rise, despite a growing adherence to the government's food pyramid. In fact, every medical study on obesity in the last ten years shows the US population steadily gaining weight - a 33% jump in the last decade alone. Now, 56% of the population is overweight, with researchers predicting that, in a few generations, every American adult will be overweight! *Hello?*

It's absolutely amazing, every American adult over-weight in a few generations! And believe it or not, all that is being offered by these researchers to fix the problem is the same old low-calorie, low-fat diets. If that doesn't work, they actually recommend stapling your stomach! It's like throwing gasoline on the fire and then complaining that the fire isn't going out.

Ultimately, my quest evolved beyond my own self-interest and became my life's mission. I quit my news job because telling people about the O.J. trial and the Oklahoma Bombing every night at 6:00 and 10:00 PM was killing my soul. What I really wanted to do was to find out what would solve these growing health problems for the greatest number of people and then tell them about that on national television.

Since I was now self-employed, unencumbered by any contract to political or corporate profit agendas (which meant no steady income in sight), I took a big breath, packed up my little blue Hyundai hatchback and drove from that small ABC affiliate in Bangor, Maine, back to California in four days so I could continue my diet and fitness investigations.

While driving, I had some time to think about the state of our national health and I actually got a little irritated. Irritated by what looked to be a stub-born refusal by the mainstream health "authorities" and government agencies to get out of denial and at least seriously question the escalating failure of their recommend-ed low-fat, high-carbohydrate diet.

You see, to many of them, if their diet doesn't work, it can't mean that there's something wrong with the diet, it must be *you* - the dieter. *You* must not be doing whatever it is they say to do strictly enough. And, if you claim you are and it's still not working, there are plenty of drugs with nasty side-effects for you to swallow to force your body into "working properly" on these low-fat, high-carbohydrate programs. Oh, brother.

Thankfully, I've also lightened up while pursuing these issues, since I had begun these studies more than a little bit outraged. It's just like my mom used to say to me for almost twenty years, as I struggled, searching for the ways to reach my own maximum human potential: *"What good is all this superhuman effort, Charlie, if your life isn't more fun!?"* And you know, she was right. Any diet and fitness program we're following should make all of our lives a lot more fun to live. Thanks, Mom.

As part of the research process, culminating in this program, I interviewed many of the nation's top medical and scientific professionals who were questioning or recommending a change from, the low-fat, high carbohydrate diet.

I also took on a few private clients, to personally guide and coach them through my program. Their success at improving their health and physical appearance has been so tremendous, that my referrals are also sent to me by a Beverly Hills plastic surgeon, who recommends my system as an alternative to liposuction.

The bottom line, and the only reason for you to keep reading this book, is that my program will work better for more of you than anything else available.

Why? Because it is the most user-friendly, genetically accurate diet and fit-ness program ever assembled. It optimizes our genetic potential, from head to toe, inside and out. Moreover, because of its straight-forwardness and unparalleled level of effectiveness, it eliminates much of the frustration and struggle that's usually associated with diet and fitness pro-grams. It is the only comprehensive program of diet, fitness and supplementation designed from our own evolutionary blueprint.

I hope you don't have to "drop dead" of cardiac arrest, suffer a plethora of health problems, almost make yourself diabetic, and struggle to lose forty pounds of insecurity-induced-fat like I did, to finally get it.

CHAPTER TWO

The Evolution Of The Diet

Human beings evolved over the last two to three million years, becoming stronger, taller and smarter, by eating the foods that were native to their environment. By the time we evolved to the point where we were most like modern humans in our behavior (about 40-50,000 years ago), there was a sudden explosion in new forms of stone and bone tools, cave paintings and artwork, as well as elaborate burials and other rituals. Not long ago, evolutionarily speaking, we lived and thrived as "hunter-gatherers," eating mostly meat, some vegetables, nuts and seeds and seasonal fresh fruits and berries. We ate eggs when we happened to get them and, depending on our location, we also ate fish.

Really? Our diet was mostly meat? Not fruits and vegetables? Yup. Loren Cordain, professor of exercise and sports science at Colorado State University, and a leader in evolutionary (hunter-gatherer) diet research puts the emphasis on "hunter," not "gatherer."

His most recent studies indicate that diets averaged 65% meat and fat (mostly unsaturated), with the rest of our diet made up of "gatherings". Completely the opposite of the USDA Food Pyramid.

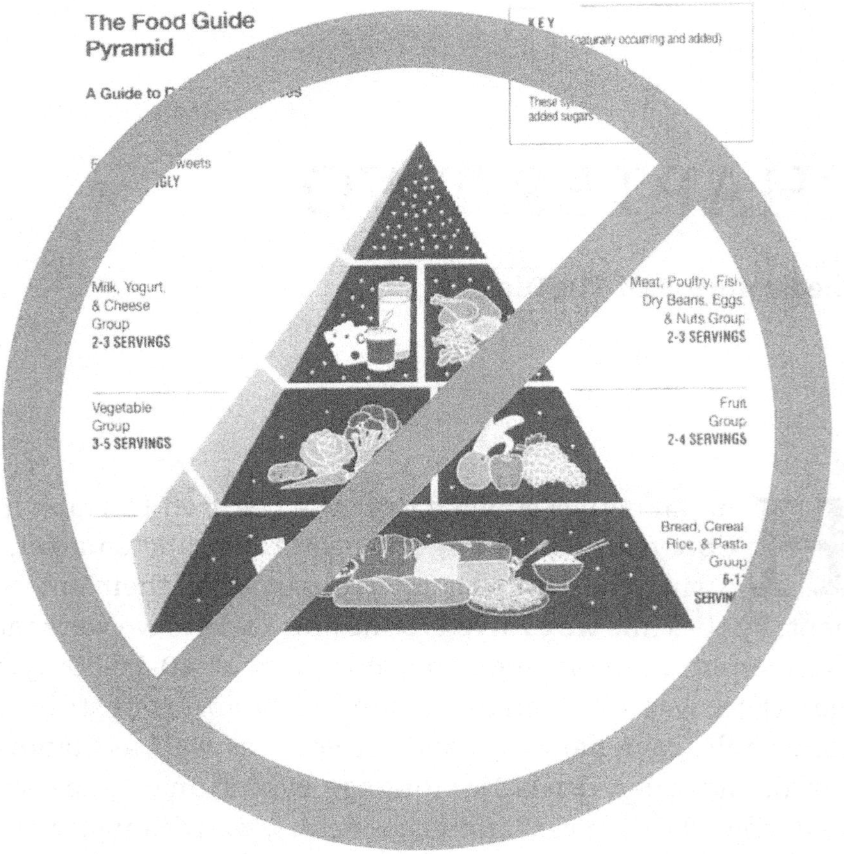

A key to understanding our dietary roots, and why it makes sense to take an "about-face" from the current low-fat, grain-based diet, is knowing what our evolutionary environment was like. That guides us towards foods that are natural for us to eat.

Our world was dominated for millions of years by multiple Ice Ages. Grains and dairy products were never part of our regular daily diet - ever. Neither were legumes, potatoes, pasta, bagels, chips nor colas. These new foods have been working their way into our diet for just a few thousand years. In the case of bagels, chips and colas, less than one-hundred years. These major shifts in our diet have resulted from the development of agriculture, industrialization, modern food processing and human inventiveness.

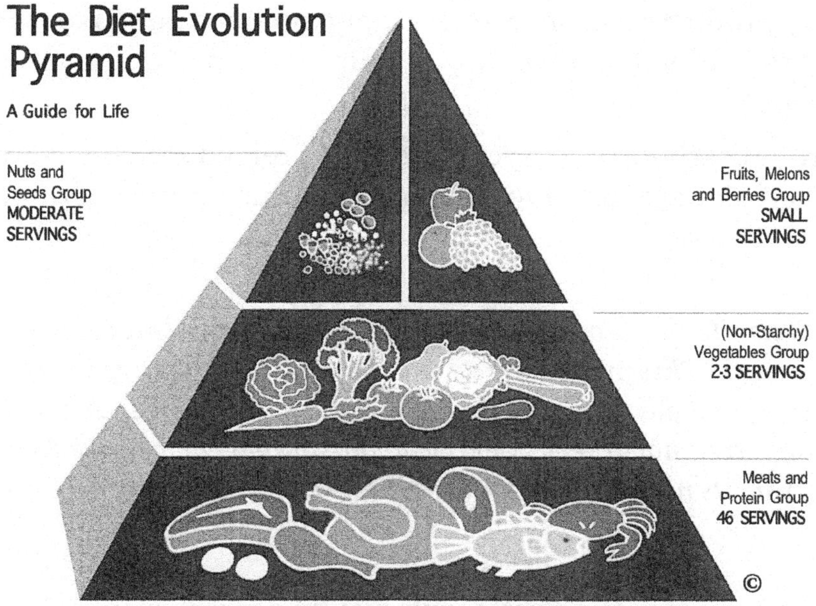

What's important to understand, and what is being missed by current mainstream diet and fitness authorities is this: no matter how wonderful this human inventiveness has been in the development of culture, science, medicine and the growth of societies, these few thousand years have not been enough time for our bodies to genetically adapt to these "new" foods. And we are paying for it with increased diseases of many kinds and a rapidly expanding national waistline. In fact, a recent CNN report: *Americans Fatter Than Ever and Getting Even Fatter* quoted a *Colorado Health Sciences Center* study: *"every U.S. adult will be overweight in a few generations,"* if we keep living and eating the way we do now.

Studies on modern-day hunter-gatherer groups, that are living pre-agricultural lives, and the archeological evidence, show the absence of most modem diseases such as heart disease, diabetes, hypertension, obesity and cancer.

It's also important to note that whenever, or wherever, "hunter-gatherers" adopted a modem diet: one high in grains, sugars, dairy products and unnatural, highly modified fats (like hydrogenated vegetable oils), they rapidly develop a host of modem diseases.

Aaron Hirschhorn, a "psycho-biology" premed student at Swarthmore College has a fun example of evolution and our diet. He says it this way:

> *"Termites love to eat wood. Most ducks are excellent at catchingfish. This make perfect sense because termites live in dead trees and ducks live near water. Natural selection shapes the digestive machinery of every organism so it can best eat food from its natural environment.*
>
> *To feed wood to a duck simply wouldn't make sense. Unfortunately, this is analogous to our current eating habits. Hundreds of thousands of years of natural selection have designed our bodies to eat the foods found in our natural habitat. Lucky Charms, pasta, and a host of other foods are simply 'evolutionary novelties."*

Recall that evolution works very slowly. Even though we're eating many new foods, our body's genetic makeup hasn't been able to keep up. The digestive machinery that we have today was designed to eat what the hunter-gatherers ate thousands of years ago.

Since this is a diet and fitness book, let me emphasize a few points that it is very important that you under-stand.

First, hunter-gatherers eating a high-fat and protein diet were not fat. And, it wasn't because they were starving between binges. All the archeological and anthropological evidence from extinct Paleolithic (Stone Age) hunter-gather groups shows that food was plentiful, not as scarce as we previously believed, and obesity was virtually non-existent.

Second, the evidence also indicates that there was no heart disease, high blood pressure, elevated cholesterol, or diabetes.

I know what you're thinking. What about air and water pollution, herbicides, fungicides and antibiotics in our food? Aren't those new toxins, that didn't exist 40,000 years ago, contributing to our ill health? Well yeah, they probably are. But the things I'm referring to, the major problems clearly threatening most of us, heart disease, adult onset diabetes, elevated triglycerides, high blood pressure and obesity, *are diet related.* The foods we eat day in and day out have the greatest effect here.

Another key factor that most diet gurus soft-sell, or don't understand, is the synergistic relationship between your appetite and your activity. What you're being told by most authorities is to predetermine how active you think you're going to be, and then to figure out how many calories you can get away with without gaining weight.

It's really much simpler than that. If you eat the foods you're genetically adapted to, the ones that are satisfying and don't leave you hungry and stressed out, your body will tell you when you've had enough. You can finally trust yourself, your body and your appetite, and you'll never have to weigh, measure, calculate or Zone "40-30-30" yourself crazy again.

Why? Because you're finally meeting your body's genetically-programmed, nutritional needs. You'll finally feel genuinely satisfied and nourished when you eat. Your appetite and your hunger is regulated by your actual activity level-not your projections of how much activity you think you're going to engage in this week. You need to know that diet and fitness are inseparable and function together to balance your food intake. No other mammal on the planet who follows their natural diet and activity patterns, eats beyond its needs.

It's also important to note that nobody binges on roast, fish or steak. Nobody binges on sticks of butter or lard by themselves. They are naturally self-limiting. When you've had enough to satisfy your nutritional needs, you stop. No problem.

Try that with sugar-grain combinations (*like cake and cookies*), sugar-fat combinations (*like ice cream and icing*) and grain-fat combinations (*like potato chips, corn chips and bread*)! We become "bottomless pits" with no natural shut-off valve. Only humans, our pets and other domesticated animals eat unnatural diets.

Where Did We Go Wrong?

Imagine the shock to our bodies 8,000 to 10,000 years ago, when our ancestors developed agriculture and switched from our normal, evolved diet of mainly meat and fresh vegetables, to a diet of mostly grains. Actually, it doesn't take much imagination-all you have to do is look around at the people in almost any public place. It is frightening to see how far we've gone astray.

As paleo- (stone age) anthropologists will tell you, wherever grains became the mainstay in human diets, there was a universal drop in height, muscularity, and even cranial capacity. Overall, health dropped significantly. In fact, archaeologists can easily tell if newly discovered bones are from a hunter-gather-er society or an agricultural one.

The hunter-gatherers are taller, have stronger, thicker bones, good teeth and are more robust than the agricultural ones.

The agriculturist's bones show rotting around the orbits of the eye, rotting teeth and extremely fragile bones.

All this when there was no polluted air and water, when soils were rich and fertile, and agriculturists were still very active.

This archeological evidence alone should cause us to rethink the food pyramid, and the false belief that grains are the perfect food-as Madison Avenue, most nutritionists and the media presently claim.

How Can We Fix It?

The problem started when our digestive mechanisms, which worked so perfectly for two million years, were suddenly trying to use unknown and unrecognized fuel, throwing our fine-tuned biochemistry into havoc. Common sense should tell us that we can fix the new problems by going back to the original diet which kept us strong, healthy and lean. Of course, this diet should be combined with enough activity that our bodies are challenged - but not trashed.

So there it is, in a nutshell *(pardon the pun)*. By eating the foods that the human body has evolved to use, and being active, we can avoid the deadly diseases of civilization and get leaner, and stronger than ever. We also significantly improve our immune system and health. Not too bad, eh?

I've simplified exactly how to do that in Part Two: The Diet Evolution.

But first, for the *"But where are your peer-reviewed studies showing that grains, and the low-fat diet are bad for you?"* ... or the *"Fat has to be bad, that's what all the magazines say!"* crowd, in the next chapter I've pulled together a few of the studies no one has shown you. And in the back of the book I've referenced a few more.

Most modern diet research is only a couple of decades old and the research constantly contradicts itself. Re-searchers change their recommendations almost every-day. Hopefully, these published studies from research organizations like the *American Journal of Clinical Nutrition, Lancet,* the *Department of the Navy,* and the *Archives of Internal Medicine* will start to calm skeptics, and hopefully help change their point of view. The research is available in Chapter Three: Death By Pyramid.

CHAPTER THREE

Death By Pyramid- The Low- Fat, High-Carb Lie

The standard view promoted by most health gurus and the encyclopedia is that fat is our enemy, and that eating fat makes us fat. Anyone who takes time to thoroughly review the available literature will quickly realize that these are ridiculously simplistic and inaccurate views. Yet a surprising number of "health professionals" still advocate these messages, continuing to mislead a fearful public, anxious to lose weight.

The low-fat diet lie is so pervasive and it's advocates so reactionary and closed off to new research and information, that noted diabetic researcher Dr. Richard K. Bernstein says:

> *"Call it the Big Fat Lie. Fat has, through no real fault of its own, become the great demon of the American dietary scene. It is no myth that one-third of Americans are overweight (authors interjection: now 56%). It is however a myth that Americans are overweight due to excessive fat consumption."*

He's not the only researcher who thinks that dietary fat has gotten a "bum rap." There's an *"avalanche of international research"* according to pediatric neurosurgeon Dr. Larry Mc Cleary, M.D., that clearly concludes that not only are low-fat, high carbohydrate diets ineffective, but that they could very well be dangerous.

The research includes evidence that low-fat diets are actually raising the risk of heart disease, diabetes, and even cancer.

For example, a 1996 study published in *The Lancet* reads,

> *"The largest and most comprehensive study on diet and breast cancer to date, studying over 5,000 women between 1991 and 1994, showed that women with the lowest intake of dietary fat had significantly higher incidence of breast cancer than women with the highest intake of dietary fat. It also found that women with the highest intake of starch had a significantly higher incidence of breast cancer than women with the lowest intake of starch. The study found no evidence that saturated fat had any effect one way or the other on breast cancer, and that unsaturated fat had a significantly protective effect against breast cancer."*

-FRANCESCHI SET. AL. INTAKE OF MACRONUTRIENTS AND RISK OF BREAST CANCER. LANCET; 347(9012):1351-61996

What this says is: *women who had diets that were the lower in fat and higher in carbohydrates had the most breast cancer!* Huh? Could it be true? The low-fat, high-carb diet followers had more cancer? That's not what we're hearing on the news everyday, is it.

Just as important, and completely counter to "low-fat logic," is this notable result from the study: saturated fat, the big dietary boogie-man that we're all going crazy trying to get out of our diets, had no effect at all. Why isn't this front page news?

If there's even the slightest chance that women are being threatened with higher levels of breast cancer by eating a low-fat diet, why are these low-fat, high-carbohydrate diets still being sold to us as the gospel and as the way to help stop breast cancer? Clearly, we should at least be following up on this kind of report, shouldn't we?

Noted lipids researcher Dr. Mary Enig, Consulting Editor to the *Journal of the American College of Nutrition* and President of the *Maryland Nutritionists Association*, says this about the low-fat lie:

> *"The idea that saturated fats cause heart disease is completely wrong, but the statement has been 'published' so many times over the last three or more decades that it is very difficult to convince people otherwise unless they are willing to take the time to read and learn what produced the 'anti-saturated fat agenda."*

More Dietary Lies- The Cholesterol Myth

> *"In Framingham, Massachusetts, the more saturated fat one ate, the more cholesterol one ate, the more calories one ate, the lower peoples serum cholesterol. We found that the people who ate the most cholesterol, ate the most saturated fat, ate the most calories weighed the least and were the most physically active."*

-FROM "ARCHIVES OF INTEMAL MEDICINE," 1992, DR. WILLIAM CASTIL/1; DIRECTOR OF THE FRAMINGHAM STUDY.

> *"The diet-heart hypotheses suggests that high intake of saturated fat and cholesterol causes heart disease] has been repeatedly shown to be wrong, and yet, for complicated reasons of pride, prof-it and prejudice, the hypothesis continues to be exploited by scientists, fund-raising enterprises, food com-*

panies, and even governmental agencies. The public is being deceived by the greatest health scam of the century."

- DR. GEORGE V. MANN, PARTICIPATING RESEARCHER IN THE FRAMINGHAM STUDY AND AUTHOR OF 1993'S "CORONARY HEART DISEASE: THE DIETARY SENSE AND NONSENSE."

There is also evidence that low-fat diets may even cause weight gain, but you never hear about that, do you?

"In a two-year study, 171 women on a low-fat diet achieved a maximum weight loss of only about seven and a half pounds at 6 months, and by year two some of that weight was regained. Most significantly, the standard deviation was more than twice the average weight loss, showing that a number of subjects actually gained weight on the low-fat diet, not counting the 13 that dropped out of the program."

- SHEPPARD L ET. AL. "WEIGHT LOSS IN WOMEN PARTICIPATING IN A RANDOMIZED TRIAL OF LOW-FAT DIETS". AMERICAN JOURNAL OF CLINICAL NUTRITION 1991;54:821-8.

As low-carbohydrate diet investigator, Dean Esmay, writes in his timely web-page essay, *The World's Biggest Fad Diet: and why you should probably avoid it*:

"Despite more than a decade of American diet gurus recommending low-fat diets for weight loss, there remains no study which clearly shows that low-fat diets result in long-term, significant weight loss among the chronically obese. In fact, most such studies show quite marginal improvements in weight, and some actually show significant weight gain among test subjects."

In addition to the studies that expose the problems with a low fat diet, interestingly enough, there are several scientists, like metabolic researcher Captain Charles Gray, MD (at the San Diego Naval Base), who studied diets that contain significant amounts of fat and low carbohydrates.

One exercise and diet study conducted at the naval base was an eye opener and raised some very interesting questions.

Before testing with humans, the first study was done with pigs, who, of all other mammals, have a metabolic make-up that most closely resembles humans.

The pig study ran twelve-weeks with two different groups. One group dieted on 7-10% carbohydrate, and 70-74% fat *(50% of the fat was saturated fat)* and the remainder of the diet was protein.

The second group used the opposite dietary composition; 7-10% fat, and 74% carbohydrate, with the remainder protein.

The animals were exercise conditioned first, tested, and a base line was established.

The results? Starting with the low-fat, high-carbohydrate group, the ones on the "healthy" food pyramid like diet, only 30% finished the treadmill test - 70% of them failed.

In the high-fat group, 80% finished the treadmill test and, on an average, ran one-third longer. In fact, the numbers should be greater because the high-fat group could have kept going longer - but the researchers tired after five hours!

Dr. Gray thinks that the pigs were able to perform this well because they were now burning fat for energy instead of sugar.

In the human study, the subjects followed a diet with the same food ratios as the high-endurance pigs: 70-74% fat *(50% of that was saturated-butter, cheese, meat)*, 7-10% carbohydrates and the rest protein.

The results? All participants' blood triglycerides (a major factor in heart disease) plummeted, 70% had their HDL (good cholesterol) increase and the LDL (bad cholesterol) decrease.

All these positive changes happened while eating over ten times the recommended amount of cholesterol.

As you can see from this small sample, and those on the following pages, there are many studies that refute the "prevailing wisdom" that high-fat diets are bad for us, and that low-fat diets are good. This "wisdom" is just plain wrong! If you want to see even more studies than the ones that follow, check out the resources and recommended reading section at the end of the book.

But the most important issue is this: **if you eat the foods you are genetically designed to eat, you don't have to fight over who's got the "right" studies or who doesn't, because your body will work the way it was designed to, perfectly.** You'll feel the difference, and you can take cues from your body instead of erroneous fads and hype.

I'm going to ask you to read the last paragraph again. I want you to understand that eating your body's genetically appropriate diet is the most important principle of the program, and is the key to trusting your own body.

What Doctors Are Saying

> *"In general, study has demonstrated that multiple risk factors for coronary heart disease are worsened for diabetics who consume the low-fat high-carbohydrate diet so often recommended to reduce these risks."*

-CHEN YD ET. AL. "WHY DO LOW-FAT HIGH-CARBOHYDRATE DIETS ACCENTUATE POSTPRANDIAL LIPEMIA IN PATIENTS WITH NIDDM?" DIABETES CARE, 1995 JAN, 18:1, 10-6

> *"The idea that saturated fats cause heart disease is completely*

wrong ..."

- DR. MARY ENIG, CONSULTING EDITOR TO THE JOURNAL OF THE AMERICAN COLLEGE OF NUTRITION, PRESIDENT OF THE MARYLAND NUTRITIONISTS ASSOCIATION, AND NOTED LIPIDS RESEARCHER

"A recent study involving over 40,000 middle-aged and older American men over a period of six years found that there was no link between saturated fat intake and heart disease in men."

-ASCHERIO A ET. AL. "DIETARY FAT AND RISK OF CORONARY HEART DISEASE IN MEN: COHORT FOLLOW UP STUDY IN THE UNITED STATES." BRITISH MEDICAL JOURNAL, 1996 JUL 13, 313:7049, 84-90

"The diet-heart hypothesis (that suggests that high intake of saturated fat and cholesterol causes heart disease) has been repeatedly shown to be wrong ... The public is being deceived by the greatest health scam of the century."

-GEORGE V. MANN, PARTICIPATING RESEARCHER IN THE FRAMINGHAM STUDY AND AUTHOR OF CORONARY HEART DISEASE: THE DIETARY SENSE AND NONSENSE, JANUS PUBLISHING 1993

"In Framingham, Massachusetts, the more saturated fat one ate, the more cholesterol one ate, the more calories one ate, the lower people's serum cholesterol ... the people who ate the most cholesterol. ate the most saturated fat. ate the most calories weighed the least and were the most physically active."

-DR. WILLIAM CASTILLI, DIRECTOR OF THE FRAMINGHAM STUDY, ARCHIVES OF INTERNAL MEDICINE, 1992

"... *evidence that low-fat diets are by and large ineffective and possibly even dangerous continues to accumulate in some of the world's most prestigious medical journals*."

-DEAN ESMAY, AUTHOR OF THE WORLD'S BIGGEST FAD DIET: AND WHY YOU SHOULD PROBABLY AVOID IT

"*We found no evidence of a positive association between total dietary fat intake and the risk of breast cancer. There was no reduction in risk even among women whose energy intake from fat was less than 20 percent of total energy intake.*"

-HUNTER, DJ ET. AL. "COHORT STUDIES OF FAT INTAKE AND THE RISK OF BREAST CANCER A POOLED ANALYSIS." NEW ENGLAND JOURNAL OF MEDICINE, 334.· (6) FEB 8 1996)

"*The commonly-held belief that the best diet for prevention of coronary heart disease is a low saturated fat. low cholesterol diet is not supported by the available evidence from clinical trials*."

-EUROPEAN HEART JOURNAL, VOLUME 18, JANUARY 1997

"*Reduced fat and calorie intake and frequent use of low-calorie food products have been associated with a paridoxical increase in the prevalence of obesity.*"

-HEINI AF; WEINSIER RL. "DIVERGENT TRENDS IN OBESITY AND FAT INTAKE PATTERNS: THE AMERICAN PARADOX." AMERICAN JOURNAL OF MEDICINE, 1997 MAR., 102(3):259-64

"*A recent American study showed that low-fat. high-carbohydrate diets (1) increase risk of heart disease in post-meno-*

pausal women over a higher fat, lower carbohydrate diet (2)."

(1) 15% PROTEIN, 60% CARBOHYDRATE, 25% FAT.

(2) 15% PROTEIN, 40% CARBOHYDRATE, 45% FAT

-JEPPESON, J., ET. AL. "EFFECTS OF LOW-FAT, HIGH-CARBOHYDRATE DIETS ON RISK FACTORS FOR ISCHEMIC HEART DISEASE IN POSTMENOPAUSAL WOMEN" AMERICAN JOURNAL OF CLINICAL NUTRITION, 1997; 65:1027-33

"A study involving tens of thousands of American women showed that diets high in carbohydrate (which almost all low-fat diets are) significantly raise women's risk of developing diabetes."

-JORGE SALMERON ET. AL. "DIETARY FIBER, GLYCEMIC LOAD, AND RISK OF NON-INSULIN-DEPENDENT DIABETES MELLI/US IN WOMEN" JOURNAL OF THE AMERICAN MEDICAL ASSOCIATION. 1997; 277:472-477

"High intake of fats from the Omega-3 group increase HDL cholesterol, which is considered protective against heart disease. Obviously, it would be difficult to eat an Omega-3 rich diet while following a traditional fat reduced diet, especially if one were following one of the popular American diets that has one eating only 20-30 grams of fat per day."

-FRANCESCHINI G. ET. AL. "OMEGA-3 FATTY ACIDS SELECTIVELY RAISE HIGH-DENSITY LIPOPROTEIN 2 LEVELS IN HEALTHY VOLUNTEERS." METABOLISM, 1991 DEC, 40:12, 1283-6. ALSO JOURNAL OF THE AMERICAN COLLEGE OF NUTRITION 1991:10(6);593-601)

"A strong correlation exists between schizophrenia and deficiencies in fats ... The possibility that diets generally low in fat might worsen schizophrenia or even bring on the condition among those already predisposed to it is hard to ignore."

-LAUGHAME JD; MELLOR JE; PEET M. "FATTY ACIDS AND SCHIZOPHRENIA" LIPIDS, 1996 MAR, 31 SUPPL:, S163-5. ALSO PEET MET. AL. "ESSENTIAL FATTY ACID DEFICIENCY IN ERYTHROCYTE MEMBRANES FROM CHRONIC SCHIZOPHRENIC PATIENTS AND THE CLINICAL EFFECTS OF DIETARY SUPPLEMENTATION." "PROSTAGLANDINS LEUKOT ESSENT FATTY ACIDS," 1996 AUG, 55:1-2, 71-5

"In addition, these studies confirm a growing body of evidence that increasing dietary carbohydrate increases plasma triglycerides and decreases plasma high-density-lipoprotein (HDL). increasing the risk of cardiovascular disease."

-METABOLISM 1993:42:365-70

"Numerous studies have shown that high-carbohydrate low-fat diets lead to high triglycerides, elevated serum insulin levels, lower HDL cholesterol levels, and other factors known to raise the risk of coronary artery disease."

-SEE LIU CC; COULSTON AM; REAVEN GM.

"EFFECT OF HIGH-CARBOHYDRATE LOW-FAT DIETS ON PLASMA GLUCOSE, INSULIN AND LIPID RESPONSES IN HYPERTRIGLYCERIDEMIC HUMANS." METABOLISM, 1983 AUG, 32:8, 750-3.

COULSTON AM; LIU CC; REAVEN GM. "PLASMA GLUCOSE, INSULIN AND LIPID RESPONSES TO HIGH-CARBOHYDRATE LOW-FAT DIETS IN NORMAL HUMANS." METABOLISM, 1983 JAN, 32:1, 52-6.

LEFSKY JM; CRAPO P; REAVEN GM. "POSTPRANDIAL PLASMA TRIGLYCERIDE AND CHOLESTEROL RESPONSES TO A LOW-FAT MEAL." AMERICAN JOURNAL OF CLINICAL NUTRITION, 1976 MAY, 29:5, 535-9.

SEE ALSO GINSBERG H ET. AL. "INDUCTION OF HYPERTRIGLYCERIDEMIA BY A LOW-FAT DIET." JOURNAL OF CLINICAL ENDOCRINOLOGY AND METABOLISM, 1976 APR, 42:4, 729-35

CHAPTER FOUR

The Twilight Of The Zone

As l write this, the most popular dietary program of the late '90s has been, according to book sales figures, Dr. Barry Sears' Enter The Zone. I remember talking with Dr. Sears during a stop on my way back from San Francisco, where I had just finished anchoring a news special for the United Nation's 50th Anniversary celebration. He was making an appearance at a neighborhood gym in the beach community of Santa Cruz, where he was promoting his ideas and a multi-level marketing company he was involved with that sold special "nutrition" bars based on his concept.

He spoke for about thirty minutes, and I found him a very interesting speaker with a talent for memorable quotes and quips. He also sounded as though he was onto something that might push us all to consider abandoning our die-hard national attachment to high-carbohydrate, low- fat, low-protein eating.

His book was, and is, however, rather technical which may be why I've never met anyone who's said they've actually finished it *(although that didn't hurt book sales).*

Let me summarize some of its main points. I'll try to make it as painless as possible and, hopefully, a little humorous. I'll also share with you the study Dr. Sears quoted publicly in Los Angeles to health and fitness professionals as proof that his "zone" program works.

More importantly, I'll share with you the part of the study he didn't bother to quote - the part that tells of a diet very similar to the *Diet Evolution* that showed itself to be six-times more effective than the "zone like" diet.

Now, I'm not here to beat up on Dr. Sears. He definitely has helped increase national awareness of how food can affect us hormonally. We should all thank him for that, and I do. Additionally, he has inspired some of us to research carbohydrate moderation and eating adequate protein - a big step in the right direction.

The Back To School Zone

The easiest parts of his book had to do with controlling blood sugar levels by eating fewer carbohydrates, and the need to eat more fat in order to bum fat.

The harder part is his new theory that forms the basis of his program: the theory of controlling *"good and bad eicosonoides"*. He says that they are the body's super-hormones, and that they control many other hormones and bodily functions. Dr. Sears thinks if you can control them, you "open the door to the zone," a state of optimum physical and mental performance. Controlling the good and bad eicosonoides requires changing our diet to a special ratio he has invented, in dietary shorthand: 40-30-30 (his secret formula).

What that ratio means in simple terms, is that we are supposed to eat exactly 40% of our daily diet in the form of carbohydrates, exactly 30% protein "not more, but not less", and exactly 30% fat.

The Oh? Zone

Progressively, the two main questions that surfaced for me about "the zone" theory were these: Were our bodies really glorified machines like cars or computers? Second, are our bodily systems so predictable, so perfectly controllable and programmable, that if we all stuck this 40-30-30 ratio of food into our mouths every time we ate, we would all function at our best?

I, being an open-minded Aquarian (is that redundant?), was willing enough to consider the possibilities. Being a practical fellow, I knew I was also out $22 + tax for the book, so I read on.

The (No) Fun Zone

Even though I was genuinely interested in Dr. Sears' theories, as I finished the beginning of the book, my mind couldn't help thinking of the first chapter of *Enter The Zone* as some kind of a nutritional horror novel. It actually was that ominous. Think something like *Dinner* by Stephen King.

For example, in the first chapter, Dr. Sears clearly states that we are to treat food as a drug. In some limited respects, he's right. A sugar or caffeine fix are clear examples of that. To think of all food as a drug, while a powerful image, is unnecessarily terrifying.

Food on the other hand, a least when it's the foods we're designed to eat, is nurturing

and nourishing, not something requiring a prescription. We should view food as our friend. We eat food. We need and require food. Growing up, we even play with our food *(and some haven't even outgrown that).*

Dr. Sears continues his drug analogy with the admonition that we must eat food in a controlled fashion *"as if it were an intravenous drip."*

I imagined Nurse Ratchet coming after me to insert lunch. *(Ouchi Quick, run!)*

The Neanderthal Zone

I also couldn't help but wonder, if this need to control our eating so strictly, like an IV. drip, were true, how fixing dinner would have been 40,000 years ago trying to eat in the proper ratio to "enter the zone" ...

> *"Our story begins late one night, 40,000 years ago. The beautiful Aggie Ogg, being very conscientious (after figuring out her lean body mass ratio), was loading a mastodon steak onto the kitchen scale to get just the right amount of protein together for dinner. Just then, Ozzie Ogg, washing a basket full of gatherings, turned to his mate and very seriously said; "Honey, how many roots and berries do we need with dinner to make 40-30-30? ... "*

Then, reading this, I was snapped back into reality:

> *" .. the rules of this dietary technology may appear complicated at first, ... (but) once you put them into practice you'll find <u>they're exceptionally easy to follow</u>."*

Hmmm ... OK. In all honesty, measuring exact percentages at every meal didn't sound so easy to me, but I wanted to give his book a fair shake. I and some of my clients gave it an honest "run for the money". But I gotta tell ya, that in my total experience with "the zone", even people I've encountered who worship it, have a lot of problems following it.

> *For example, my clients, which include world class athletes who are exceptionally disciplined, "entered the zone" alright - the constantly complaining, stressed-out, "I screwed up again", dieting mentality zone.*

Evidently my clients are not the only ones who have run into these difficulties because it's taken the publication of three more books to try to explain to his readers how easy it is to follow his program; *Master The Zone, Zone Perfect Meals in Minutes* and *Zone Food Blocks*.

And now, for the next time you're in the kitchen with your PC or MAC, following his program is so darn easy there's even a *Zone Manager* computer program you can buy to *"make menu preparation a snap!"* Gee, sounds really easy to me. Go figure.

But have no fear. When you see how simple it is to follow the *Diet Evolution* style of eating without the requirement of diet-scales, multiple books or computer programs to figure it out, you'll finally be able to relax and enjoy your meals while getting the results you want.

The End Zone

To date, Dr. Sears doesn't have any scientific studies to prove his theory. When the question of scientific proof came up at a talk to professional athletes and trainers at the Hyatt Sunset in Los Angeles, he quoted a dietary study published in the *American Journal of Clinical Nutrition (Golay, et al, Geneva University Hospital, AJCN 1996; 63:174-8)* that showed a diet similar to his, which, when compared to the assumed "healthy" diet showed an 8% improvement in insulin levels. This, he said, was *"statistically significant"*, proving that his diet worked.

> *But Dr. Sears didn't bother to quote the part of the study that tells of a diet very similar to the Diet Evolution that showed itself to be* ***six-times more effective*** *than his "zone like" diet.*

The other diet in this study used two-thirds fewer carbohydrates *(15% of daily intake)*, than the "zone like" diet *(45% carbohydrates)*.

The results of the 15% carbohydrate diet? You might say they were statistically significant too. It showed a 46% improvement in insulin levels vs. an 8% improvement from the "zone like" diet? That's almost six-times more effective at lowering insulin - the body's fat-storing hormone.

The study also said that blood sugar levels, cholesterol and triglycerides all *"decreased significantly in the 15% carbo-hydrate diet"* but *"neither insulin nor triglycerol concentrations fell significantly"* in response to the "zone like" diet.

Needless to say, the *Diet Evolution's* principles are in accord with the 15% carbohydrate diet.

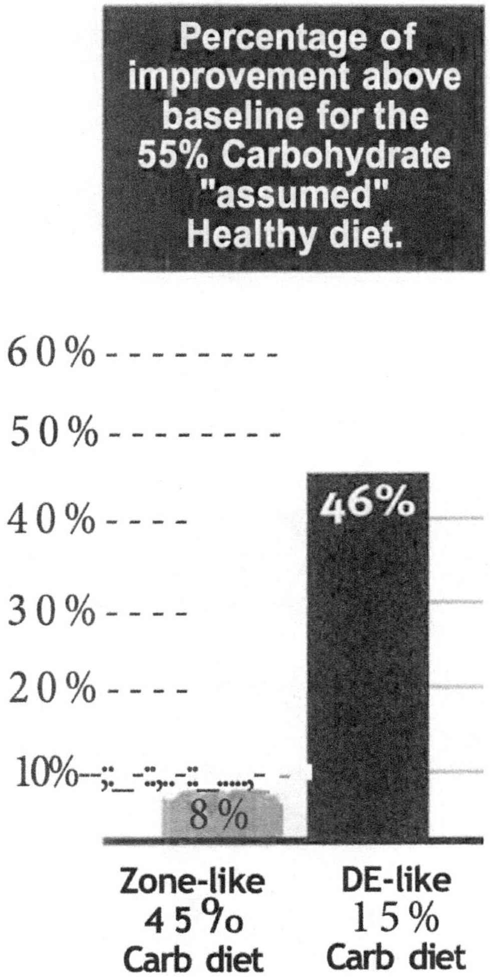

So what's the secret formula? **The real secret is that there is no secret formula.** There is no new theory. And thank good-ness there is no 40-30-30. There is just physical anthropological fact.

The closer you can come to basing your current diet on the foods our ancestors evolved with and thrived on for thousands and thousands of years, the easier it will be for you to become lean and healthy.

And ultimately, eating right is incredibly easy to do. Not just a little easier, *a lot easier*.

CHAPTER FIVE

Diet Evolution Vs. The Popular Diets

- ❖ The Zone's 40-30-30
- ❖ Atkins dieting
- ❖ Low-fat, high carbohydrate with aerobics
- ❖ Low-fat, high-carbohydrate with weightlifting

Other diet programs have proven to be far too complicated. For example:

• eating at five pre-set times a day

• long form journaling

• measuring every ounce of food

• counting calories

• estimating fat grams

• calculating protein needs by approximating activity levels and lean body mass

Ultimately, they all fail to become comfortable lifestyles because they oppose our bodies and minds natural design and rhythms. They completely ignore over 2.3 million years of human development. Up until about 8-10, 000 years ago, almost all of us were lean, vital & strong, much like our modern-day Olympic athletes. All of these other programs focus on short term goals, not long-term solutions.

How Is Diet Evolution Different From Barry Sears' "40-30-30" Enter The Zone?

• no complicated "food blocks"

• no unrealistic laboratory like "ratios" every time you eat.

• no unnecessary and unnatural fear of food.

• not inconsistent and confusing. Zone recipes use foods that contradict his diet recommendations

• food is a not drug needing to be *"controlled like an IV drip"*

How Is Diet Evolution Different From Dr. Atkins' "Low-Carbohydrate" Diet Revolution?

• DE doesn't unnecessarily raise carbs to stop ketosis

• no counting grams of carbohydrates necessary if you eat from the DE basic foods list

• no "controlled portions" of modern domesticated foods that are the most common allergens, addictive, and promote fat storage. DE returns you to instinctual "control" - you can trust your body, and your food, again

• fitness is as important as the eating plan

How Is Diet Evolution Different From Susan Powter's "Low-Fat, High Carb" Give Me Five? (Infomercial)

This style of daily aerobics, lack of strength training and eating a food pyramid diet:

• gradually cannibalizes lean body mass

(so you do *"shrink, shrink, shrink"*)

• increases body's ability to make fat (compensation)

• suppresses testosterone

• suppresses growth hormone

• suppresses the immune system

• People on such diets are dogged by hunger, and over-eat carbohydrates to compensate. This diet elevates insulin, promoting fat storage. It also elevates triglycerides, setting the stage for coronary heart disease.

Many researchers now say low-fat diets are actually dangerous, contributing to disease *(see Chapter 3, Death by Pyramid).*

How Is Diet Evolution Different From Larry North's Great American Slim Down? (Infomercial)

• old body builders "pre-contest" diet repackaged

• too many carbs & low fat

• even highly motivated body builders have difficulty following this kind of program and are notorious for binge eating after a diet cycle

• you have to eat every three hours-because you're so hungry it's the only way to stay on it

• this program violates its own principles by making, cheese, pizza, and macaroni and cheese, proteins!

• The small print says to use "fat-free" cheese, but users are not in control over that except at home, and they are being taught to think of these foods as "proteins" in general.

• Additionally, fat-free cheeses don't melt well and taste horrible.

• Body builders can get themselves to do almost anything in the short term to get ready for a competition, but regular folks will balk at the compromises in taste and texture of fat-fee substitutions.

• And finally, the infomercial workout tape doesn't take the user through an actual program.

PART TWO: A NEW YOU

The Diet Evolution

6 Get Ready to Start
7 Keeping Track
8 DE Overview
9 Basic Food List
10 Meal Suggestions
11 Supplements
12 Why Diets Fail
13 Eat Fat and Get Fit FAQ

CHAPTER SIX

The Diet Evolution

Get Ready To Start

Put a calendar on the front of your refrigerator, a wall in your kitchen, or in your home office where you can easily see and mark it every day.

• Take two sets of "before" pictures from the front view, side view, and back view, and get two sets made when your film is developed. You should wear snug fitting clothes such as gym shorts and t-shirt, bathing suit, or form fitting pants and shirt. Keep one set and mail the other set to me with your short bio within the next 48 hours.

• Tape one of your new photos to the top right-hand side of your program calendar. New "progress" photos should be taken every six-weeks. Tape the sixth week photo below your first on the right side of your program calendar.

• Take your *Basic Foods* and *Suggested Meals* lists to the store with you and stock up on your favorite foods from this list.

• Circle the day you start on your program calendar, and six weeks from that date.

• Post your *fitness self-test* next to your program calendar and fill in the blanks with your scores.

Test yourself again at 6 and 12 weeks. Cut out and fill in your chart (see page 61).

CHAPTER SEVEN

The Diet Evolution

Keeping Track

Boldly cross-off each day on your program calendar in which you've followed your new diet & fitness program to your satisfaction.

This is a simple way to see, "at a glance," how you're doing.

Seeing all those days checked-off back-to-back is a great motivator (right slash [/] for diet, left slash [\] for fitness).

CHAPTER EIGHT

The Diet Evolution

Overview

Humans were not designed to eat certain foods
Our human genes, formed by millions of years of evolution, are a bad match for today's grain-based and highly processed modern diets.

Eat the wrong foods and the body malfunctions, eventually making us fat, sick, devitalized, impotent and unhappy.

Eat the right foods and we can quickly maximize our genetic potential.

"How To" Summary:

1. Eat only from Charles' *Diet Evolution* Basic Foods list. (a)

2. Eat whenever you're hungry. (b)

3. Don't count calories, or fat grams. (c)

4. Don't weigh, measure or keep a diet diary.

5. Be active following Charles' fitness program guide-lines.

6. Supplement with Charles' Essential Fatty Acids, Anti-oxidants and Vitamins. (d)

7. Drink plenty of pure water *(coffee or tea, cream OK)*.

(a) These are whole, natural foods that will spoil; meats, vegetables, fruits, nuts and seeds.

(b) Primarily natural fat and protein combinations.

(c) Hunger is self-regulating in response to activity

(d) Dr. Eades recommends extra potassium (99 mgs.) with each meal while in your fat loss phase

CHAPTER NINE

The Diet Evolution

Basic Foods List

Eat naturally-raised meat, including:

beef, lamb, pork, veal, game, organ meats, rabbit, all fish, seafood, chicken, duck, quail, pheasant, and eggs to your satisfaction.

Eat a variety of fresh, non-starchy vegetables:

preferably organic, uncooked, in salads, lightly steamed or stir-fried, and in soups made with homemade meat stocks from the bones of chicken, beef, lamb or fish to your satisfaction. *(meat stocks great for sauces too)*

Eat only traditional fats and oils including:

animal fats *(lard)*, extra virgin olive oil, expeller pressed sesame oil, flax oil and the tropical oils. *(coconut and palm)*

Eat fresh, raw nuts, seeds and nut butters.

(moderate amounts)

Eat a variety of fresh fruits and berries.

(preferably organic, small amounts)

CHAPTER TEN

The Diet Evolution

Meal Suggestions

Breakfasts

Steak and eggs *(my favorite!).*

Eggs; poached, scrambled, omelet or frittata style.

(with favorite non-starchy additions; bacon, avocado, any hard cheese, chives, herbs, tomato, chopped veggies, salsa, spinach, salmon, any meat, fish or poultry. Top with sour cream if you like)

Lox, eggs and onions. Fried, sunny, over-easy. Benedict style.

(without the muffin)

Any meat, fish or poultry you would care for as breakfast is OK too.

Salmon, or sliced turkey rolls, w/cream cheese OK if you tolerate dairy. (good for lunch or snack too)

SMALL side of whole fruit, berries or melon. *(no juices)*

H20, coffee, tea. *(no sugar)*

Lunches & Dinners

Appetizers-salads, soup such as gazpacho w/sour cream.

Meat plates.

Shrimp grilled or chilled w/ garlic butter or mayonnaise. *(no red sauces)*

Artichoke w/butter/mayonnaise.

Mixed green or garden salad. *(any no-sugar-added dressing)*

Main meal Caesar salad with double portion of chicken or salmon. (no croutons)

Any grilled, broiled, baked meat, fish or poultry. *(watch out for flour in sauces)*

Grilled/steamed non-starchy vegetables.

Desserts- Berries. *(with heavy cream if you want, whipped if no sugar only)*

When in Doubt, Keep it Simple

Garden salad with olive oil vinaigrette. *(no sugar dressing)*

5-6 oz. protein-beef, chicken breast, turkey or favorite fish.

(baked, light grilled, broiled, light stir-fry, poached-no breading)

Large portion of steamed vegetables. *(non-starchy)*

8 oz. or more of appropriate beverage.

½ cup fresh berries.

CHAPTER ELEVEN

The Diet Evolution

Supplements

Vitamins, Antioxidants & Essential Fatty Acids

We need fewer supplements following the Diet Evolution program because the foods listed in the basic foods list, supply higher amounts of the known, and unknown, nutrients our bodies need every day.

It's important to note that grains interfere with the absorption of many nutrients. On a diet without grains, less supplementation is necessary.

Similarly, when you follow the program, you won't be ingesting the artificial elements found in the highly processed, modern foods normally found in the *Standard American Diet.*

Supplementation to fight off those artificial elements is therefore less in need.

With supplements, the best idea is to take the ones that reflect what we understand about the nutrient composition of our evolutionary past, and the ones that we know can protect us from modern deficiencies and pollution.

I recommend going to your local health food store (or now,

Amazon) and get:

1. a broad multi-nutrient vitamin and mineral.

2. essential fatty acids (EFA) or DHA in capsule form.

3. an anti-oxidant formula made by any major manufacturer.

4. a ninety-nine mg. potassium supplement (99mg.), to take with meals *during initial dietary transition*.

CHAPTER TWELVE

The Diet Evolution

Why Diets Fail

Lyle McDonald, certified strength and conditioning specialist, says that people who do the most poorly in terms of weight loss/weight maintenance share the following patterns.

1. Excessive caloric deficits.

A trainer had a 180 lb. women whose nutritionist put her on 800 cal/day. End result was no weight loss in 1 year. If you're on a calorie counting diet *(trainer's rule of thumb)*, eating 12 cal/lb. works well to start, but can be adjusted up or down as necessary. If you follow the DE program you didn't need to count calories.

2. Too little, or too much exercise. Both are bad. Too little exercise and you get nothing, too much and you slow your metabolism down just as with too few calories. Moderate exercise, no less than 3 hours per week is the minimum that yields any results. Most people do well on 4-5 hours per week.

3. Insufficient protein and fat.

The RDA for protein is insufficient and certain fats are essential. 1 gram of protein per pound of body weight should be the standard intake. Weight training increases protein needs.

4. Too many modem carbohydrates.

Even evolutionary carbohydrates should average no more than 15-35% oftotal intake.

5. Only want a quick fix.

They drop a lot of weight very fast and always gain it back. Deliberate changes are easier to maintain for life than extreme dieting.

CHAPTER THIRTEEN

The Diet Evolution

Eat Fat And Get Fit!

Frequently Asked Questions (FAQ)

When I coach clients in the principles of the Diet Evolution, there are still a few questions that come up more than any others. The reason questions still persist in the minds of a lot of people is that most "health reporters," who ought to check into the facts, don't do their homework and, unfortunately, keep perpetuating outdated findings. I recently spoke with Michael Eades, M.D., who, along with Mary Dan Eades, M.D., runs *The Colorado Center for Metabolic Medicine* in Boulder, Colorado. We both found that our clients had the same questions about our pro-grams.

Almost everyone readily accepts the common sense of returning to our genetically determined foods, but we've all been assaulted by one-sided, low-fat, high-carbohydrate reporting for so long, that it's reassuring to hear from a physician schooled in the principle that most of us will be much healthier returning to our genetically-appropriate diet.

Before we look at the most frequently asked questions, let me emphasize that if you're a type-one diabetic, have kidney disease, or any other serious illness that you're under care for,

PLEASE SEE A PHYSICIAN WHO UNDERSTANDS AND HAS EXPERIENCE WITH THESE PRINCIPLES, or consult the Eades at *The Colorado Center for Metabolic Medicine in Boulder*, before making significant changes to your diet. The following answers are from Dr. Michael Eades.

#1 I'm sure I can lose weight on this diet, but will it cause me to have a heart attack because meat will raise my cholesterol level?

That's simply not the truth and actually quite the oppo-site because of the underlying biochemistry that's involved. When you eat a low-carbohydrate diet you actually lower your body's production of cholesterol. The majority of cholesterol comes from your body's own production, not from your diet.

#2 Will this diet cause osteoporosis?

The theory is that when you eat protein, it's broken down into substances that are a little bit acidic. Supposedly, this leaches the calcium out of the bones, and can give us osteoporosis later on.

This sounds logical, but just doesn't happen. Researchers found that when people eat a lot of protein-especially meat protein, they don't have any increase in urinary calcium. In other words, they're not leaching calcium out of their bones and losing it in their urine, as the theory would imply.

In fact, when we look at the skeletal remains of hunter-gatherers who ate two-to-three times the amount of protein considered "safe" for us today, you find their bones are 17% more dense than ours - when comparing individuals of the same height and sex.

A recent article in *The American Journal of Clinical Nutrition* relates the risk of hip fracture to diet. The strongest correlation to non-fracture is animal protein. Eating a diet high in meat actually strengthens the bones!

#3 Will this diet damage my kidneys?

No - this is a long-standing medical myth. In fact, it has been shown in multiple studies that eating more protein will not damage normal kidneys in any way. One study compared the normal age-related decline in kidney function of vegetarians *(eating a low protein diet)* to body builders *(who ate a large amount of protein)*.

The study showed essentially no difference in the rate of decline. In other words, protein consumption has no effect on the normal decline of kidney function.

#4 Is saturated fat a problem?

Based on my personal experience with clinic patients I don't think it's a big deal-saturated fat is pretty much harmless. It's not particularly biologically active and all it does is get stored, or it gets burned. There are a number of studies correlating the intake of saturated fat with HDL *(good cholesterol)* levels. The people who ate saturated fat had higher good cholesterol levels. The people who shifted to diet lower in saturated fat had lower good cholesterol levels.

If saturated fats have any bad effects, whatever they might be, they seem to be neutralized by a low-carbohydrate diet, like DE, or another evolutionary type *(no grains)* diet.

#5 I've heard that low-carb diets cause rapid weight loss of water only. Is this true?

No - low-carbohydrate diets such as this reduce blood pressure very quickly. It does that by causing diuresis *(increased production of urine)*. It does this because most people eating the *Standard American Diet*, or a low-fat hi-carb diet, are already retaining too much fluid. So, at the beginning, the program simply gets rid of excess fluid, and then they lose primarily fat.

It's not uncommon in our medical practice to have patients losing 100-150 lbs. Unless they were water balloons there's no way that the excess was just water.

#6 I just started the program and I've been feeling a little tired. Why is that?

This is not uncommon at first. It takes a little time for your stomach's enzymes to adapt to a lower-carbohydrate diet. I always tell my patients not to do anything too strenuous for a few days-until they adjust to the new diet. When your body does adapt, you'll have more endurance and you'll feel a lot better.

Patients sometimes feel like they're "out of gas" in the first few days. If you feel that slump, or you feel hungry, don't try to solve it by going out and eating carbohydrates. You'll just set yourself back.

If you're going to eat, eat extra protein and fat such as any kinds of nuts or seeds *(not peanuts-they're a legume, like a bean)*, sliced meats, leftover meats, hard boiled or deviled eggs. These are all good alternatives to get protein and fat into your diet to give yourself a little pick-me-up without disrupting your dietary transition.

#7 Will I lose weight faster if I cut out carbohydrates completely? And would it be dangerous?

Actually, it wouldn't be dangerous at all. There are many societies that thrive without carbohydrates in their diets - Australian Aborigines and Eskimos are two examples.

Human biochemistry is designed to do very nicely with-out carbohydrates, but if we go without proteins we will die. If we go without fat we die - not as quickly as we do if we don't get protein, but we die nevertheless.

If we don't get carbohydrates, nothing happens. And that's why it doesn't make sense to go on a high-carb diet at the expense of fat and proteins.

As far as losing weight more quickly, you may lose a little faster, but you'd be missing out on some of the important phytochemicals and antioxidants we find in plants that we need to be truly healthy. Eating only meat can get a little boring.

#8 Why are fruits limited during fat loss, and fats not limited?

The amount of fruit is limited because it tends to raise insulin *(the fat storing hormone)* more than the other food on the program. If you think about it, our hunter-gatherer ancestors would have never eaten fruit on a daily basis, because it was only available seasonally. Fat, on the other hand, doesn't stimulate our body's production of insulin.

I don't want to give you the impression that fats are completely unlimited-to lose weight, you have to limit incoming calories at least to a level that creates a deficit between what you're eating and what you're using. But in truth, fats are so satisfying to the appetite, your body will usually limit its intake. Just be sure they're good quality fats-nut and seed oils, olive oils, animal fats, butter - not trans-fats or hydrogenated fats like margarine.

#9 Are nuts really a healthy food choice?

Yes - nuts are a good portable choice of high-quality fats and protein, available to us since hunter-gatherer times. True nuts, such as almonds, macadamias, pistachios, pecans, walnuts, pinons, Brazil nuts and cashews, all offer a healthy source of calories.

Use nuts to snack on, or add to foods. They are an especially good snack when you are at your desired body weight. You should only eat small to moderate amounts if you want to lose body fat.

Do not eat peanuts though, remember they are not really nuts at all but legumes, and are more likely to stimulate allergy problems. Peanuts are also too high in carbohydrates.

#10 What about the Chinese? Don't they eat a lot of rice and have lower heart disease?

If you look at the latest statistical abstract from the *American Heart Association* (published in the Feb. 1999 edition of *The American Journal of Clinical Nutrition)* that compares the rates of heart disease by country what you find out is that rural Chinese men and women have lower rates of heart disease than American men and women. But the *American Heart Association* doesn't differentiate between rural and urban Americans.

When you look at the urban Chinese their rates of heart disease are about the same as the American average. In fact, the womens' are even greater.

If you "buy" into the idea that elevated insulin levels are a major risk factor for heart disease, which just about everybody does, whatever you can do to get insulin levels down can prevent heart disease.

Look at the three ways that keep it down. The main thing is restricting carbohydrate in the diet. You can also keep insulin down by exercise, or a low-calorie diet in general. The majority of rural Chinese work very hard and eat a low-calorie diet. Even though there's more rice in their diet, they still keep their insulin down because they work so hard and don't eat that much.

That's why marathon runners and exercise addicts can get by on vegetarian-type diets. These people exercise like crazy, then the minute they quit exercising they gain weight.

PART THREE: FITNESS

Diet Evolution Fitness

14 Getting Started
15 Self-tests
16 Introduction
17 Back to the Basics
18 Beginners Program-Overview
19 Beginners Home Program
20 Intermediate & Advanced Programs-Overview
21 Intermediate & Advanced Programs

CHAPTER FOURTEEN

Diet Evolution Fitness

Getting Started

A) A recent physical by a licensed physician is recommended.

B) Complete the easy "current fitness & progress" self test.

Cut-out self-test chart on page 61, and post next to your calendar. These are five simple at-home tests, to record on your chart. They'll help show your current fitness level and personal progress in relationship to the optimal range.

You'll test the four physical factors that affect fitness levels: *Aerobic condition, Strength, Flexibility, and Body-Fat.*

Please re-test yourself and update your records at 6 weeks and 12 weeks.

C) Take your Starting Photos.

Take them again at 6 weeks and 12 weeks- front, back and side view - in snug clothing or a bathing suit.

CHAPTER FIFTEEN

Diet Evolution Fitness

Self-Test

Record your scores on your chart (page 61)

#1 Aerobic Conditioning

1.5 Mile Endurance Test. It's best to do this at your local high-school or college running track.

Warm up by walking at an easy pace for two or three minutes. Start at one end of the field and time yourself with a stopwatch, or wristwatch with a second hand.

Start your watch and begin walking as fast as you can. Give it your best, but if at any time you feel dizzy, sick or weak - stop immediately!

If you prefer to have a supervised test, your local YMCA may have an appropriate program to assist you with. When you finish the 1.5 miles (6 laps around a standard track), stop your timer and write down your time to the nearest second on your chart (see page 61).

If this seems like it's too far for your conditioning level, just pick any distance that you can time and repeat to use as a benchmark, and time yourself against that distance.

#2 Push Ups (Upper-Body Strength)

Men, do as many full-pushups as you can. Women, do as many knee or full push-ups as you can. Record the number you do on your chart.

Full push-ups are done by lying on your stomach with your palms on the floor directly in front of your shoulders. Push your entire body up off the floor so you're balanced on your palms and toes, then lower yourself back down to the floor. To avoid injury, be sure to tighten your stomach and keep your back flat.

Knee push-ups are done by lying on your stomach with your lower legs lifted off the floor, ankles crossed. Push your entire body up off the floor, but you will be balanced on your palms and knees, not your toes. Lower yourself back down to the floor.

#3 Crunches (Abs and Lower Back Strength)

Lie on your back with your arms crossed over your chest, palms in the center. Curl your head, neck and shoulders up off the floor, "crunch" style.

This is not a full sit-up, only as far as you can go before you lift your upper body off the floor towards your knees. Do as many as you can without pausing and write that number on your chart. If your back hurts doing this test, don't do this one.

#4 Sit and Reach (Legs and Lower Back Flexibility)

Put a 12-inch piece of masking tape on the floor. Take a tape measure lay it across the masking tape at the 15-inch mark so that they cross each other and form a cross. Sit down with your legs straight out so that your heels are touching the masking tape, and the 15-inch piece of the measuring tape is extended out away from your feet. Take a breath and, as you exhale, stretch forward as far as you can comfortably.

Repeat this three times and write down how far you reached forward *(on the tape measure)* on your chart.

#5 Percentage of Body-fat

Do this one just for fun. All body-fat tests are notoriously inaccurate for a host of reasons, but most folks want to try it out any way. Using the charts below and on the following page to check your percentage. Follow the directions below the graphs on pages 59 and 60. All you need is a ruler!

And please, don't get hung up on the body-fat percentage mania.

Remember, you are not a percentage of body-fat. You are an amazing living being, with innumerable, irreplaceable qualities that can't be defined or measured.

For both Women and Men: your relative body-fat measurement is at the point where the ruler crosses the "percent fat" line.

Women: Use a ruler to line up your hip measurement with your height.

For example: if your hips measure 36.5" and you are 5'2" tall, then your body fat is about 26%.

If You're a woman, use this chart

BODY-FAT PERCENTAGE CHART FOR WOMEN

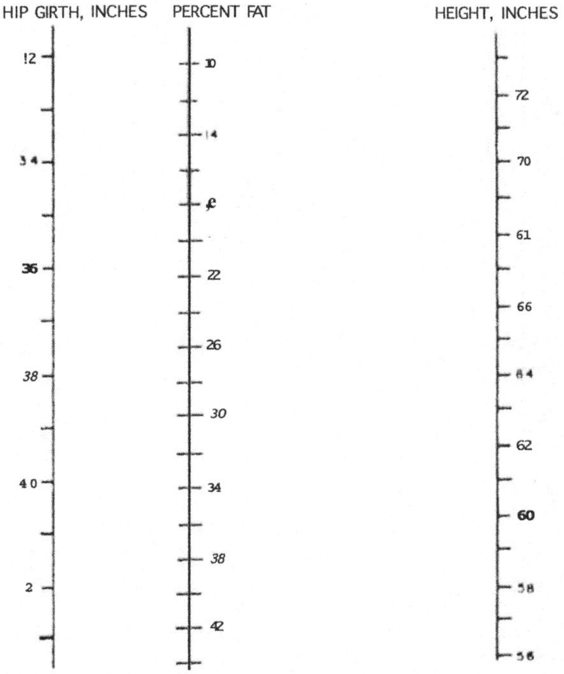

From *Sensible Fitness* (p.31) by J.H. Wilmore, Champaign, IL: Human Kinetics Publishers. Copyright© 1986 by Jack H. Wilmore. Reprinted by permission

For both Women and Men: your relative body-fat measurement is at the point where the ruler crosses the "percent fat" line.

Men: use a ruler to line up your waist measurement with your body weight.

For example: Men, if you weigh 170 lbs. and your waist is 34", then your body fat is about 18%.

If You're a man, use this chart

BODY-FAT PERCENTAGE CHART FOR MEN

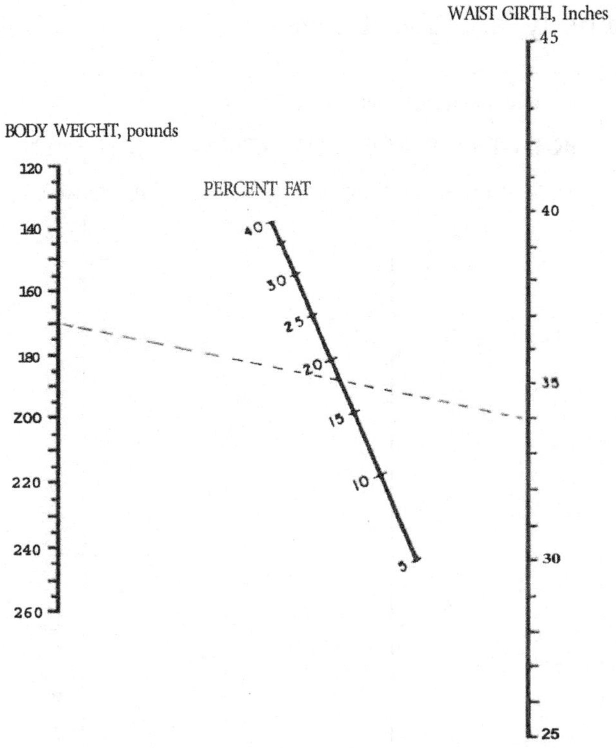

From *Sensible Fitness* (p.31) by J.H. Wilmore, Champaign, IL: Human Kinetics Publishers. Copyright© 1986 by Jack H. Wilmore. Reprinted by permission

Self-Test	Day 1	6 Weeks	Optimal Score
Aerobic Conditioning			18 minutes or faster
Push-ups			23 or more reps
Crunches			40 or more reps
Sit and Reach			19″ or more
Body-Fat Percentage			Men: 12-20%
			Women: 16-20%

CHAPTER SIXTEEN

Diet Evolution Fitness

Introduction

- Developing the major muscle groups that give us shape, tone, strength, and burn fat.
- Even small increases in daily activity can drastically increase overall health.
- Studies show that metabolic rate goes up by approximately 35-40 calories for every pound of muscle gained.

Weight bearing fitness training, along with the *Diet Evolution* food plan, keeps you from losing muscle, adds new muscle, keeps your metabolic rate strong, and increases fat loss in both men and women. If anything, this effect is more pronounced in women, because they are starting with less muscle mass *(generally)* than men and have more to gain from it.

If you're new to fitness - start out with just a little exercise and build up as your tolerance increases, or you can break it up into 2 or 3 short sessions in the same day and get roughly the same results. At every level, feeling challenged, but not trashed, is what we're after.

CHAPTER SEVENTEEN

Diet Evolution Fitness

Back To The Basics

• Three days a week are "getting strong" days and three are aerobic/play days.

• More advanced folks can jump ahead to the appropriate level after the first two weeks of following the *Diet Evolution* food plan. This means very moderate exercise, even for the highly advanced, during dietary transition.

• Challenge yourself wisely by using the *"Rating of Perceived Exertion"* scale. Simply rate each exercise from "1" (1 being sitting on the couch) to "10" *(10 being maximal intensity).* When you're first beginning, aim for a rating of 4 *(very light).* Then, over the first four weeks, gradually bring up the intensity of each exercise. For example, this might mean a few more pounds on the weight training exercises or a few more minutes of aerobic/play.

By the end of 4 weeks you should be doing pretty well on the strength days.

According to legendary fitness guru Jack LaLane, and *Certified Strength and Conditioning Specialist* Lyle McDonald (CSCS), most people will triple their first day's results in this short period of time. And for people who have been very unfit, this is unbelievably motivating.

Additionally, most of you should be able to do thirty-minutes of aerobic/play activity by the end of these first four weeks too. If you have the time available to do more as you feel stronger, go ahead and do more, just be sure to mix-up your intensity levels (hard for a few minutes, then easy for a few-then repeat).

For beginners, this: strength-then play pattern, continues for the second four weeks (thirty-minutes of strength training 3x a week and thirty-minutes aerobic/play 3x weekly).

This is only three-hours of exercise per week, occasionally more, if you are doing more aerobic-play.

Beginners move from home to gym workouts at week 8 to 12. This allows you to use greater weights safely, and adds an environment of camaraderie.

For intermediates, we use the same pattern, but move from home workouts to the gym if you can after the first four weeks.

For intermediates that want to continue at home, just increase the number of sets, and slow the movements down to increase intensity.

Lyle McDonald, CSCS, shared on the Internet the improvements he sees when training beginners:

> *"Women are always amazed when they start lifting. For example, they may be using 5 lb. dumbbells in the bench press and struggling. Telling them that they will be lifting the 15 or 20's (pound weights) by the end of 8 weeks usually gets rather incredulous looks from them. But the feeling of accomplishment they experience when they do it about 8 weeks later is wonderful to see.*
>
> *This translates into a big difference in quality of life, especially for older individuals who may have lost a lot of strength and muscle. My Mom was impressed that she could take out*

the garbage or the recycle bin by herself."

Lyle and I also enthusiastically agree that these kinds of results and responses are why we love strength training so much. In the beginning stages, untrained individuals make instant progress, clearly getting better from workout to workout. You get fast, positive feedback, which is critical to the success of what you are trying to accomplish.

CHAPTER EIGHTEEN

Diet Evolution Fitness

Beginners Program Overview

What You'll Be Doing

All strength days start with a 10-minute warm up (walking for 6 minutes, easy stretching for 4 minutes) Wear loose, comfortable clothing.

Most of the exercises use your own body weight to begin with, so no weights will be needed.

Beginners First Strength Day

Every woman I've coached wants great legs, hips and buns, and the guys need more lower body strength to power them through their activities, so that's where we'll start.

I'll also write the descriptions of each exercise in easy to understand language, instead of trying to "wow" you with the medical dictionary. You'll look just as good after you've done these if you're thinking about the back of your leg when you're doing them, instead of thinking about your hamstring.

Day one will be four different exercises doing one "set" of each; door handle squats (buns), front leg raises (front of the leg), heel-to-butt raises for the back of the leg (ham-strings) and side heel raises (hips). This takes about five-minutes: only 10-15 minutes total including the warm-up and a cool down with stretching at the end.

If you don't already know how, great stretching programs are available from the YMCA, health clubs, physical therapists, chiropractors, or Bob Anderson's *Book of Stretching.*

Goals:

- 10-12 repetitions
- watch your form
- easy breathing and controlled speed
- easy stretching for flexibility to finish up

Beginners First Aerobic-Play Day

Everyone starts out easy. Goal: 10-15 minutes, 20 minutes maximum choosing from the aerobic/play list suggestions; moderate walking, stationary bike, recumbent bike, low-impact aerobics, free-form dancing or rebounding.

Depending on your fitness level, some of you might go 20 minutes from the outset, but everybody stops at 20 minutes. Each workout adds a little bit more, stretching for flexibility to finish.

Beginners Second Strength day

You'll start with the four exercises from the first workout and add three new ones; calf raise (calves), abs (stomach) and lower back. Add 3-5 repetitions to the exercises from the first workout. It will be easier by the second workout. Stretching for flexibility to finish.

Beginners Second Aerobic/Play day

Add a few more minutes of aerobic/play of choice at a low intensity.

Beginners Third Strength day

You'll add the final three strength exercises for a total of 10 different exercises that condition all of your major muscle groups for all-around conditioning. This takes about twenty minutes when you're only doing one set, plus, stretching for flexibility to finish.

In week two, beginners increase to two sets, or continue to build repetitions.

In week three, beginners increase to 3 sets.

In week four, beginners work to maximize 3 full sets.

At week five, Intermediates conditioning at home can switch to the advanced pattern at the gym with additional exercises.

CHAPTER NINETEEN

Diet Evolution Fitness

Beginners Home Program

First Strength Day

All strength days start with 10 minute warm up (6 mins. walking, 4 mins. easy stretching). Wear loose, comfortable clothing.

Most of the exercises are body weight only to begin with-no weights.

Four different exercises- "one set" each.

#1 Door handle squats (buns).

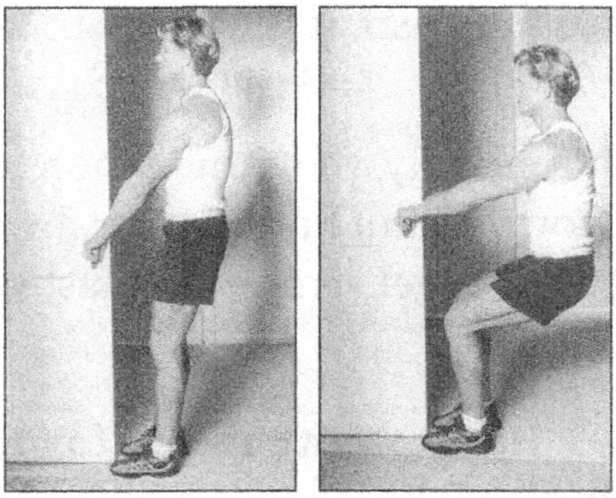

Open a sturdy door into a space that has nothing in your way. Face the outer edge of the door (see photo), stand up straight and hold firmly onto the handles, place both feet squarely under you, shoulder width apart.

While maintaining a firm grip on the handles, squat down as if sitting onto a chair. Stop when your upper legs are level with the floor, and them push yourself back up with your legs.

Continue repeating this movement 12 times without stopping. When you're finished with those 12, that's "one set" of the exercise. Now, move on to #2.

#2 Front leg raises (front of the leg).

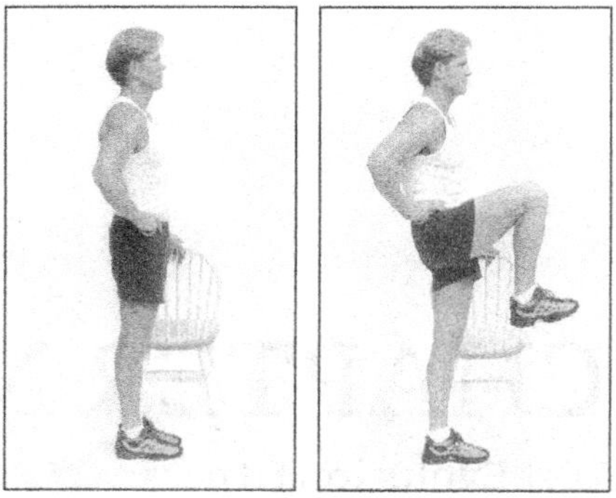

This is really simple, but you'll get great results. Stand next to the back of a strong, sturdy chair *(or you can hang onto the kitchen counter, or a desk top).* Hold your stomach in and be sure not to lean forward. Start with the right leg, and lift it slowly up towards your chest as far as you can go. Now, lower (don't drop) your leg back to the floor. Do the same movement with your left leg slowly lifting towards your chest, and then lowering it back down - that's "one repetition" because you have to work both legs to complete the full exercise.

Now, repeat the right and left leg lift eleven more times. It's easy to keep track of two - sided exercises if you count in *"one and"* style.

As you lift your right leg it's *"one"*, then as you lift your left leg it's *"and"*. So, it'll be easy to keep track as *"one-and ... two-and ... three-and ...* " all the way to twelve.

It's exactly the same when you are working your arms. Don't worry if you find the last few a little harder to do at first, these muscles get strong very fast with regular use.

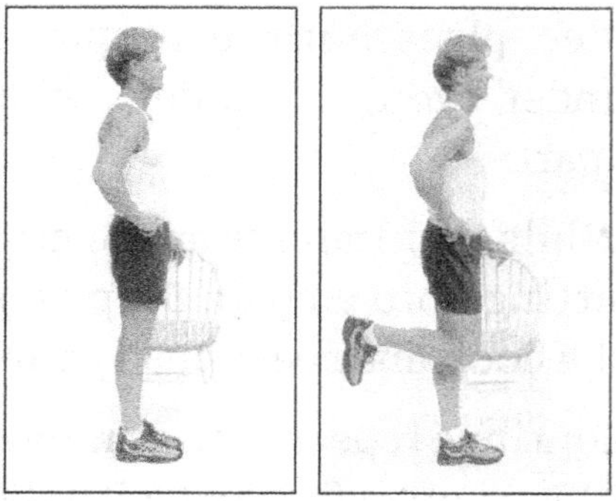

#3 Heel-to-butt raises for the back of the leg (hamstrings).

This time, stand facing the back of your chair and slowly lift your right heel up as far as you can towards your butt. Slowly lower it back down, and then, do the same thing with your left foot. Remember to count in *"one-and"* style, and repeat the movement 12 times.

#4 Standing side-leg raises (hips).

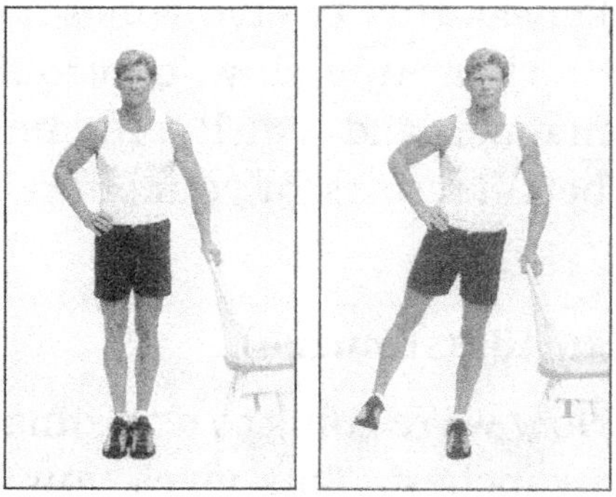

Now, turn side-ways to your chair, just like you did for your front and rear leg raises. Keeping your body straight, lift your foot straight out to the side as far as you can go without bending at the waist *(see photo)*. Do this twelve times, then turn around and do the other side exactly the same way.Finish up by doing some easy stretching. That's it for your first strength day! Congratulations!

First Aerobic-Play Day

Remember to start easy. Today's goal is to go about 10 to 15 minutes choosing from these aerobic/play suggestions; moderate walking, stationary bike, recumbent bike, low-impact aerobics, free-form dancing or rebounding.

Depending on your fitness level you might go up to 20 minutes from the outset, but no one should exceed 20 minutes. Stretching for flexibility to finish.

Second Strength day

First, you'll start with the four exercises from your first workout. Add a few repetitions to each exercise if you weren't able to do twelve the first time. If you did, you can go up to fifteen repetitions on each to challenge yourself a bit more. Now we'll add these three new ones: calf raises, abs, and lower back.

#5 Calf raise (calves).

Stand straight up facing your chair *(a desk top or counter top is O.K. too)*. Place your feet shoulder width apart and push up onto your toes. Hold for a moment, and lower your-self back down.

Repeat this twelve times, and do them in a slow, controlled manner and you'll see much better results for your effort.

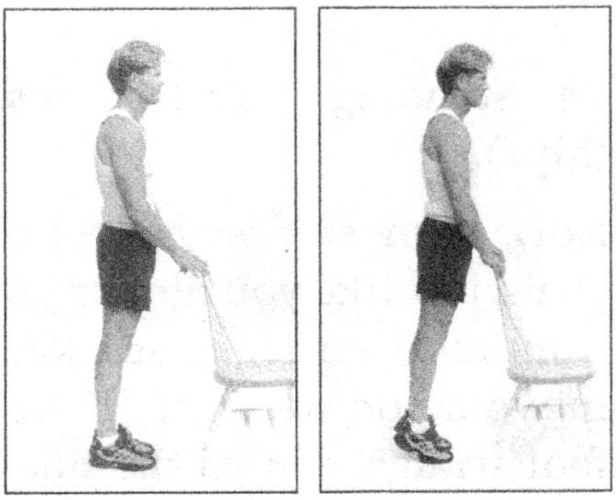

#6 Abs (stomach).

Now we're going to do stomach "crunches". This gives you all the benefits of those expensive ab-rollers, without the risk of injury or the hassle of fooling around with unnecessary equipment.

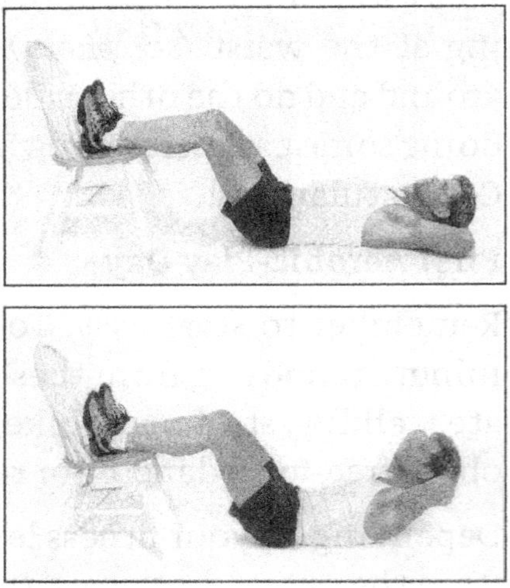

Lie down in front of your chair on a soft surface (carpet, thick towel, or mat). Facing up, place your feet on the seat of the chair, lace your fingers together behind your head (see photo), and rest your head in your hands.

Slowly, keeping your hands behind your neck, pull yourself up towards your feet, focusing on pulling from the center of your chest as if a string were tied to your breast bone, and you were being pulled up from there.

Don't worry about sitting all the way up. Only top athletes are strong enough to do that. All you need to do is pull with your stomach muscles and not from your head. It's a little tricky at first, but it gets easier very fast.

#7 Lower back.

It's often said in sports training circles that 75% of your strength lies between your knees and your chest. This is why it's so important to strengthen your stomach and back muscles- they support everything you do, every move you make, everyday.

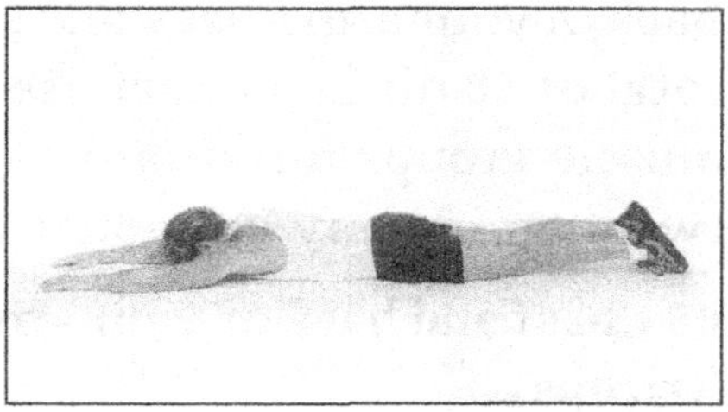

For this one, lie face down on a clean, soft surface. (You may want to place a towel under your face too.) Stretch your arms out over your head as far as you can reach and tighten your buns to protect your back.

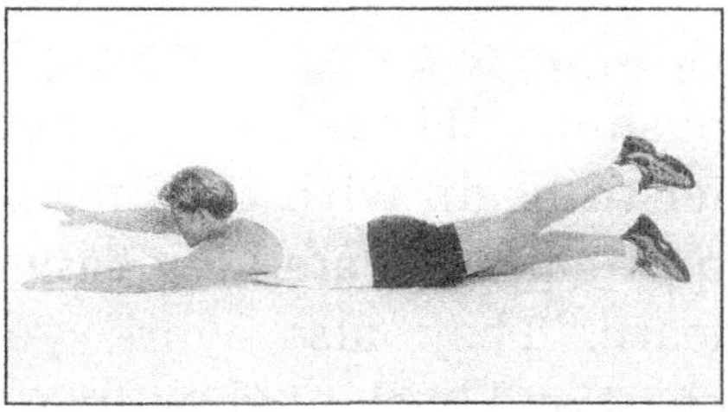

Now lift both your arms straight up as high as you can and hold them for a moment, then relax and lower them back to the floor. Repeat this twelve times.

Now, keeping your arms extended over your head but on the floor, lift your feet straight up towards the ceiling, just like you did with your arms. *(This may be a little harder at first, but you'll get the hang of it after a few tries.)*

Repeat this one twelve times too.

As you get stronger you can mix this one up by lifting your right arm and left leg at the same time, holding, and then relax.

Repeat this with your left arm and right leg too. (See photo) Then, when your stronger, you can lift both arms and both legs at the same time! That's a pretty tough version, but you'll get there soon.

Finish up with easy stretching for flexibility.

Second Aerobic/Play day

Add a few more minutes of aerobic/play of your choice at a low to moderate intensity.

Third Strength day

Today we'll add the final three strength exercises: chest and back of your arms, back and shoulders, and front arms. This is a total of 10 different exercises that condition all of your major muscle groups for all-around conditioning. This takes about twenty minutes when you're doing one set.

#8 Chest and back of your arms (triceps).

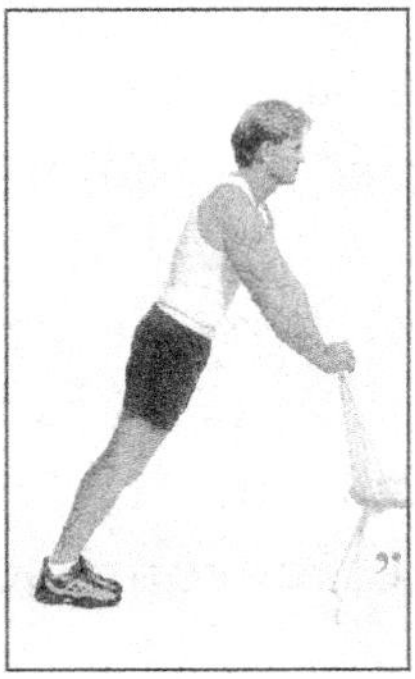

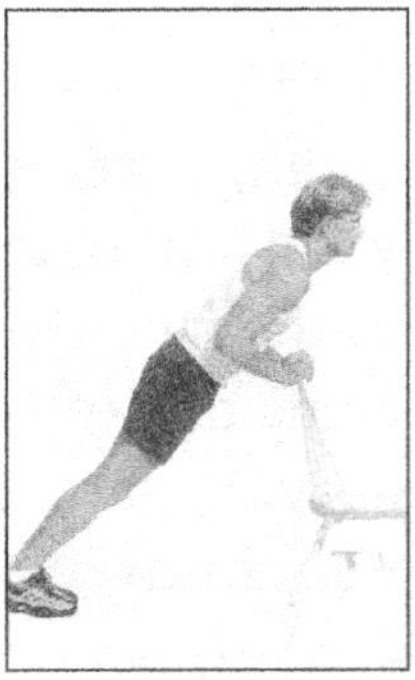

Now we're going to do angled push-ups. These are much easier to begin with than regular push-ups, and are very easy to learn. They also work your chest and back of your arms at the same time.

Stand facing the back of your chair. You can also do these against a wall, or desk top to change the angles and work different parts of your muscles. *(The wall position will be the easiest, then the chair and finally the desk)* Hold on firmly and lower yourself down towards the chair, desk, or wall *(see photos on opposite page)*. Then simply push yourself straight back up, keeping your elbows close to your sides. Once you've mastered these variations you may want to try regular face down push-ups too, just to mix it up.

<u>Caution: Make sure if you're using a chair that it's on a surface that it will grip so it won't slide out from under you!</u>

#9 Back and Shoulders

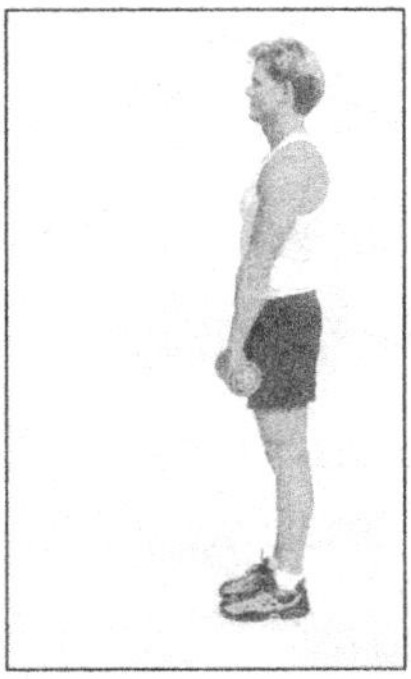

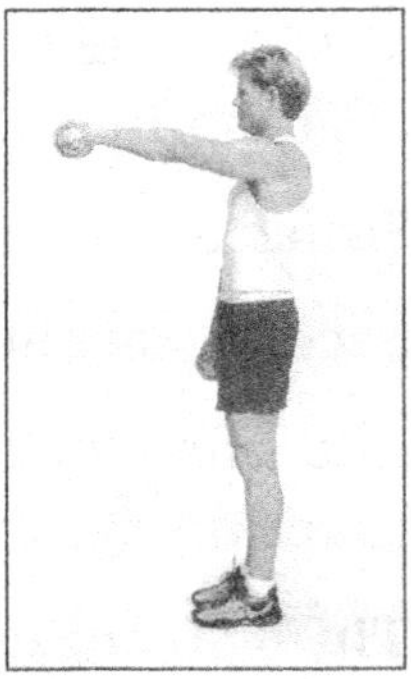

Lets start with standing front dumbell lifts for your back. Using a light pair of dumbbells that you can get at any sporting goods store *(1-3 lb. each to start)*.

Stand straight up and let the dumbbells hang at your sides, palms facing back. Then lift one dumbbell at a time straight up to shoulder height, and then lower it slowly back down (see photo).

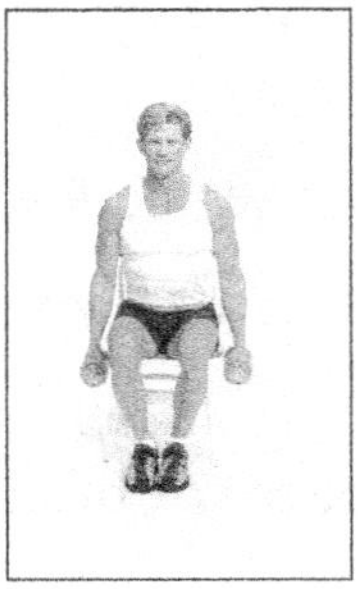

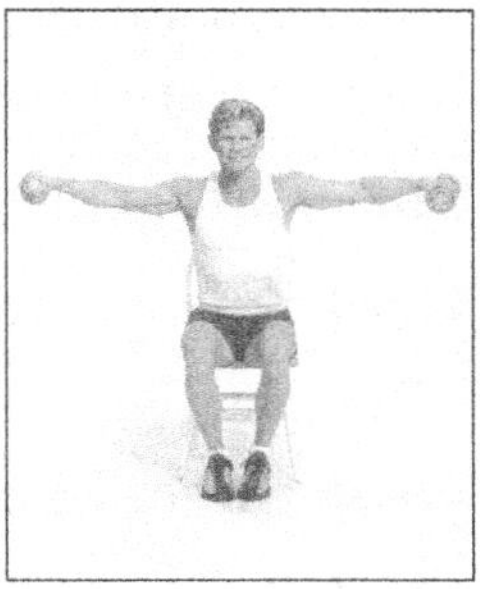

Repeat with the opposite arm, counting in *"one-and-two-and ... "* style for twelve repetitions. You can also start with soup cans if you don't have dumbbells available.

Now, we'll work the shoulders. Keep your dumbbells with you, sit down in your chair *(keeping your back straight)* and let the dumbbells hang at your side, palm facing in.

This time lift both arms straight out from your sides at the same time, stopping at shoulder height *(see photo)*. Hold for a moment, and slowly lower them back down. Repeat this twelve-times if you can.

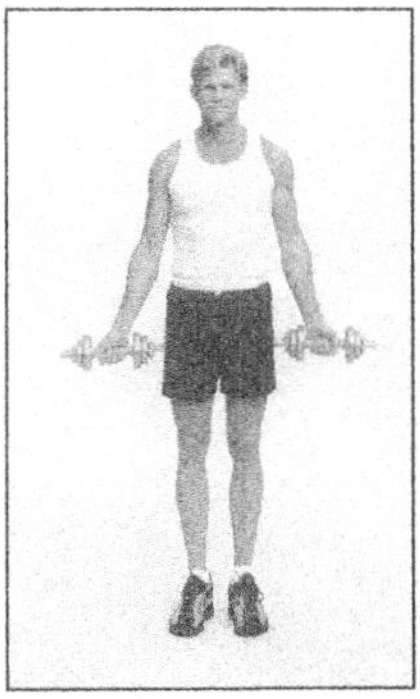

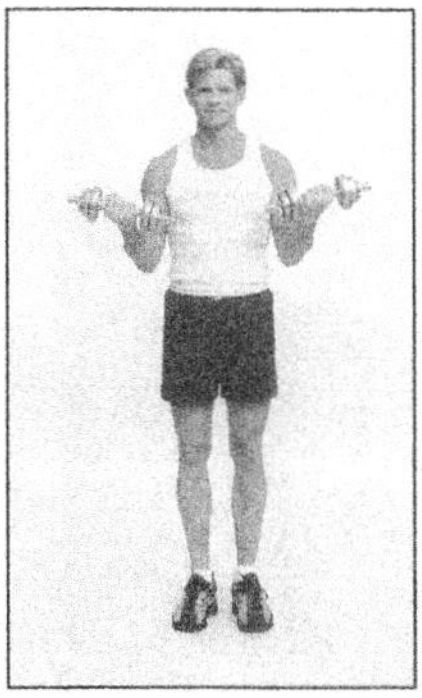

#10 Arms

For arms, we'll do standing dumbbell "curls". Stand straight up and let your dumbbells hang straight at your sides, palms facing out.

Now, one arm at a time, lift the dumbbell *(or soup can)* straight up towards your shoulder, keeping your elbow at your side. Repeat with the other arm, slowly lowering it back down to your side.

If this is not difficult for you, you can lift both arms at the same time, being sure to keep your elbow in at your side *(see photo)*.

That's "one set" of everything. Congratulations! Do your easy stretches to finish.

Third Aerobic/Play day

Add a few more minutes of aerobic/play of your choice at a low to moderate intensity.

That's it for the first week. Relax and enjoy a day off!

Week two - increase to two sets, or continue to build repetitions.

Week three - increase to three sets.

Week four - work to maximize 3 full sets.

At week five, Intermediates who are conditioning at home can switch to the advanced pattern, preferably at a gym, with additional exercises.

CHAPTER TWENTY

Diet Evolution Fitness

Intermediate & Advanced Programs

Overview

Note: *All advanced strength days must be done in a gym environment*

Summary

For most active people, starting the advanced program will consist of cutting back on: the number of workouts, the time spent in the workout *(40 minutes maximum)*, and the number of sets *(pushing up the pace and intensity a bit)*.

At every level, feeling challenged, but not trashed, is what we're after.

Getting Strong days: Monday, Wednesday, Friday

One upper body day, focusing on large muscle groups.

One lower body day, focusing on large muscle groups.

One overall day, focusing on balanced proportions.

Aerobic-Play days: Tuesday, Thursday, Saturday

Goal - build up to 30 minutes at various intensities

Suggestions: Rollerblading, bicycling, power walking, racquetball, swimming, tennis, basketball, brisk hiking, mountain biking, sprint-walks *(not jogging or running)*, rebounding, dancing.

CHAPTER TWENTY-ONE

Diet Evolution Fitness

Intermediate And Advanced Programs Detail

By now you should be at your local gym. See a staff member for any questions you have about your form while performing the exercises. Each exercise should be done in two to four sets at a time.

Monday- Upper body

12 minute aerobic warm up *(recumbent bike, efx, power-walk on treadmill)*

CHEST

- Bench Press

- Incline Press

- Decline Press

BACK

- Forward and Reverse Lat pull downs

- Bent-over rows

SHOULDERS

- Behind the neck press

- Upright rows

- Dumbbell shrugs

- Lateral raises *(side, front, back)*

ARMS

- Barbell curl & Triceps dumbbell kickbacks
- Dumbbell curl & Triceps press downs
- Scott curl & Triceps kickbacks
- Wrist curls (forearms)

ABs

- Crunches
- Vertical knee raises (roman chair or hanging knee to chest)

12 minute aerobic warm-down & Flexibility Routine

Tuesday- Aerobic/Play

Wednesday- Lower Body

12 minute aerobic warm up (recumbent bike, efx, power-walk on treadmill)

LEGS

- Squats
- Hack squats
- Leg extension
- Leg curl

CALVES

- Crunches
- Vertical knee raises- Standing calf raises *(3-ways)*
- Seated calf raises *(3-ways)*

ABs

- Crunches
- Vertical knee raises

12 minute aerobic warm-down & Flexibility Routine

Thursday-Aerobic/Play

Friday- Symmetry Day

Work the areas you see you need a little more to bring out the look you want.

12 minute aerobic warm-down & Flexi-bility Routine

Advanced level II

For the major jocks among us, follow this schedule

Upper Day

Aerobic-Play

Lower Day

Aerobic-Play

Symmetry Day

One "Off Day"

Add another Aerobic-Play day.

PART FOUR: RECIPES

Diet Evolution Recipes

Introduction

Most of the following recipes were originally shared on the internet by folks from all over the world who are following these evolutionary dietary principles.

They wanted to help each other find tasty, interesting meals, snacks, and modifications of familiar favorites. All of the recipes that follow, fit into their new lifestyles. These folks are committed to helping each other stay on track, which is sometimes a challenge in today's grain and sugar-based food culture.

Setting up your kitchen is a breeze because all you need are your favorite spices and your normal utensils. Most modern kitchens have a blender. You can use a coffee grinder to grind herbs and nuts. If you want to make your own meat jerkies, you'll need a good food dehydrator.

Shopping is even easier. Just take your basic food list to the store with you and stock up on your favorite fresh foods from each section of the list.

Most stores are set up with all the basic foods around the outside of the store - produce *(vegetables, fruits, nuts & seeds)*, deli counter *(prepared meat salads, sliced meats)*, meat department *(beef, lamb, veal, pork, fish)*, and dairy *(as a condiment!)*.

You'll almost never need anything from the inner food aisles as most of the food there is over-processed, sugared or made from grains. Spices, pork rinds *(to replace chips and croutons)*, frozen fruits and vegetables, coffee and teas are the main exceptions to the *"inner-aisle"* rule.

When you're in a hurry, need quick snacks, or you are too busy at work to get away, stock up on deli-prepared chicken and tuna salads, most stores have several varieties *(just check for that there are no added sugars or potatoes)*.

Don't forget sliced turkey and roast beef, deviled eggs, and raw *(unsalted)* nuts and seeds. Almond, macadamia and cashew nut butters are great snacks with celery sticks or sliced cucumber, and many stores carry them now *(health food stores for sure)*.

<u>Don't forget to eat whenever you are hungry,</u> and enjoy the new variety of healthy fat and protein foods that you've been avoiding for too long.

Each recipe is presented in the contributor's own words with full credit. Many, many thanks.

These recipes should give you more than enough ideas to keep your meals interesting and fun.

If you would like to have the opportunity to share your own meal, snack or dessert ideas with others, please send them to de_recipies@seizethedaymedia.org

Recipes submissions should be grain-free, dairy-free *(or opional)*, potato and bean-free.

Bon Appetit!

BEEF

Infallible Rare Roast Beef

(This really works!) 1 roast beef, with or without bones, ANY SIZE. In the morning, preheat oven to 375°F. Put roast in and cook for 1 hour. Turn off heat. Leave roast in oven. Do not open door. Thirty minutes before serving, turn oven back on to 375°F. If you need the oven for something else, take it out to "rest" and cover with aluminum foil. Every slice is uniformly pink and gorgeous. The first few times you do this takes courage!

From Barbara Baxter in "3 Rivers Cookbook"

Lemon Pot Roast

2-1/2-pound chuck roast

1 1/2 cup water

1/2 cup lemon juice

1 onion, chopped

1 teaspoon salt

1 teaspoon celery seed

1 teaspoon onion powder

1/4 teaspoon black pepper

1/4 teaspoon marjoram, ground

1 each garlic cloves, crushed

3 slices lemon

Put roast in a shallow pan or marinating container. In a medium bowl, combine remaining ingredients. Pour over roast. Cover, refrigerate at least 4 or up to 24 hours. Remove roast from marinade, place in a roasting pan. Cover and bake at 325°F. 1 1/2 to 2 hours, or until ten¬der when pierced with fork.

From: rec.food.recipes archives; Adapted by Patti Vincent

Steak Pizzaiola Ala Rick

4 beef strip steaks, cut 1/2 inch thick,

6-8 ounce each 3 tablespoons olive oil

1/4 teaspoon pepper

1 small onion, chopped

2 garlic cloves, chopped

2 teaspoons chopped fresh oregano or 1/2 teaspoon dried

pinch of hot pepper flakes

1 14 ounce can Italian peeled tomatoes, drained and chopped

[You can combine everything several hours ahead of time and heat just before serving. This is best on the barbecue, with grilled veggies.] Pound steaks between 2 pieces of wax paper or plastic wrap until flattened to 1/4-inch thickness. Brush with 1 tablespoon oil. Season with pepper In a non-reactive medium saucepan, heat the remaining 2 tablespoon oil over medium heat. Add onion and cook 2-3 minutes, or until softened. Add tomatoes, oregano, garlic, and hot pepper flakes. Bring to a boil, reduce heat to low, and cook 7- 8 minutes to blend flavors. Cover and keep warm. Light a hot fire in grill, or preheat broiler. Grill or broil steaks 3 inches from heat for 2 minutes. Turn and cook 1-2 minutes ore, be careful not to overcook. Serve with sauce spooned over the meat.

From "36'5 Easy Italian Recipes" by Rick Marzullo O'Connell

Yum Num Tok-Thai beef salad

Sirloin steak, grilled and sliced about 1/4" thick

Chopped red onions (you can sauté these if you don't like raw onions)

Cilantro, chopped Scallions, chopped Hot oil

2 or so dried hot peppers, crushed 2 tablespoons lime juice

Grill the steak. Let cool; slice. Chop onions and sauté if desired. Let cool. Add to steak. Chop cilantro, scallions. Crush hot peppers; add to hot oil. Add lime juice. Mix everything together and serve over a bed of lettuce. The Thai style beef and onion salad I had at another restaurant had crushed nuts (probably peanuts) sprinkled on top, but I think slivered almonds, lightly toasted, would be just as good.

From Mara <lindo@RADIX.NET>

Grilled Steak With Provincial Herbs

4 Natural Gourmet Steaks 1 tablespoon Olive oil

2 Garlic cloves, minced

2 teaspoons minced fresh rosemary or 1 teaspoon dried, crumbled 2 teaspoons minced fresh thyme or 1 teaspoon dried, crumbled

2 teaspoons minced fresh basil or 1 teaspoon dried, crumbled Fresh ground pepper

Place steaks in shallow dish. Rub both sides with oil, garlic and herbs. Add pepper. Let stand 1 hour. Prepare barbeque (high heat) or preheat broiler. Cook steaks 2 inches from heat source to desired <loneness, 4 minutes per side for rare.

From: The Madonna Inn in San Luis Obispo.

BEEF, GROUND

Hans' Meatballs

1-pound ground meat (I have used both elk and beef

1 medium carrot

1 small onion (including green stalk is best)

1 egg

spices as you wish

Finely grate the carrot, chop the onion in a food processor and then pour in the other ingredients. Mix. Make into small balls (the mix is quite wet and loose, so this could get messy). Fry-Enjoy.

From Hans <hans-k@ALGONET.SE>

Just Plain Chili

2 pounds of lean ground beef 1 bell pepper

6 cloves garlic

2 tablespoons olive oil

fresh ground pepper to taste

3 tablespoons cumin, or to taste

1 1/2 tablespoons chili powder, or to taste 1 can tomatoes (28-32 ounce)

Light coals in grill. While coals are setting, 30-45 minutes, form ground beef into large patties. Clean, de-seed, and chop the pepper. Mince garlic. In a large deep-shouldered skillet, heat olive oil, milling in fresh pepper to taste. Add bell pepper and sauté 5-7 minutes. Turn heat off and stir in minced garlic. Grill patties over coals until medi¬um rare, no more than 5 minutes on each side. Turn heat on high under skillet and place patties in skillet with garlic, oil, and pepper mixture. Break up patties into small pieces with spatula and brown meat thoroughly. Add tomatoes. Mash and break up toma¬toes with spatula, and mix in thoroughly. Add enough water to cover all ingredients, reduce heat to low, and let simmer 2 hours or more.

From "Jack's Skillet" by Jack Butler.

Steak Tartar Or Cannibal Canapes

4 pounds fresh ground round steak

2 cups finely chopped onions

1 cup finely chopped parsley

3-ounce jar of capers pepper to taste

Mix ingredients together, pack into a bowl. Cover and let stand in refrigerator for 1 hour before serving. Turn upside down on a plat¬ter to serve. From Mrs. Edward D. French in "Seasoned in Sewickley" Casual Joe Brown and crumble some ground beef with chopped onions and garlic (about an onion to a pound or a bit more of beef.) Pour off the excess grease, stir in a package of chopped spinach, cooked and well drained. Then stir in 3 or 4 beaten eggs, and stir until eggs are set. I don't even like spinach and I love this dish!

From Dana <dcarpend@kiva.ne!>

Sloppy Joes

1-pound ground beef

2 tablespoon. olive oil

1 medium onion, chopped

1 medium green pepper, chopped

2 cloves garlic, minced

2 cups tomato sauce

1 tablespoon chili powder

1/2 teaspoon cumin powder

Add to the pan:

1-pound ground beef, crumbled

Sauté onion, green pepper, and garlic in olive oil until tender. Continue cooking and stirring until the beef starts to brown (make sure beef is crumbly). Then stir in tomato sauce, chili powder, cumin. Let simmer for a few minutes. Serve wrapped in lettuce or by itself.

De Correct Meat Loaf

Using your favorite meatloaf recipe, substitute cabbage for bread or oats. I mix all my spices, egg, onion etc. into the meat first. Then chop up the cabbage (about a half head) and mix that into the meat mixture, then bake. It's good with Ray's Barbeque sauce mixed in it too.

From Patty <garyv@PR!MENET.COM>

VEAL

Osso Bucco/Roasted Veal Shanks

6 pieces veal shanks, each about 2 1/2 inches long 3 tablespoons olive oil

2 tablespoons lemon juice 1/4 teaspoon pepper

1 onion, cut up

3-5 tablespoons hot water

Place veal in single layer in heavy roasting pan. Sprinkle with oil, lemon juice, and pepper. Arrange onion on top. Cover and cook in 350°F. oven for 1 1/2 hours or until tender. Uncover and brown for 30 minutes longer, adding water to increase natural juices, if necessary. This recipe can be used with a veal roast. Substitute shoulder or rump roast for the shanks and proceed as above.

From Kathie Bernstein in "The Great tomato Patch Cookbook"

Veal, Carrot And Chestnut Ragout

18 fresh chestnuts-If fresh chestnuts are unavailable, roasted vacu¬um-packed chestnuts-sold in jars in the specialty foods section of many supermarkets-can be used.

2 1/2 pounds veal stew meat, cut into 2xl-inch pieces 4 tablespoons olive oil

1 1/2 cups chopped onion

1 1/2 tablespoons chopped garlic

1 bay leaf

2 1/2 cups canned low-salt chicken broth

3/4 cup dry white wine

6 medium carrots, peeled, cut into I-inch pieces 3 tablespoons chopped fresh sage

Preheat oven to 400°F. Using small sharp knife, cut an X in each chestnut. Place in roasting pan. Bake until tender and shells loosen, about 35 minutes. Cool slightly. Remove hard shell and papery brown skin from each nut. Set nuts aside.

Pat veal pieces dry with paper towels. Sprinkle with pepper. Heat 2 tablespoons oil in heavy large pot over medium-high heat.

Working in batches, add veal to pot and cook until brown on all sides, about 10 minutes. Using slotted spoon, transfer veal to large bowl. Heat 2 tablespoons oil in same pot. Add onion, garlic and bay leaf. Reduce heat to medium; cover and cook until onion is tender, stirring occasionally, about 5 minutes. Stir in broth and wine. Add veal and any accumulated juices from bowl. Bring to boil. Reduce heat. Cover; simmer 45 minutes, stirring occasionally. Add carrots to stew. Cover and cook until carrots are almost tender, about 25 minutes. Uncover and cook until meat is very tender and liquid is reduced to thin sauce consistency, about 25 minutes longer. Stir in nuts and sage. Simmer until nuts are heated through, about 3 minutes. Discard bay leaf. Transfer ragout to bowl. Serves 6.

Italian Veal Chops

8 veal chops pepper to taste oregano chopped parsley

2 garlic cloves, minced

1 can (1 pound 12 ounce) tomatoes

In skillet, brown chops. Season with pepper. Sprinkle with oregano and parsley. Add garlic and tomatoes. Cover and simmer until tender, about 2 hours.

From Vivian Kelly in "The Great Tomato Patch Cookbook"

Veal Roast (Arrosto)

2 garlic cloves, minced 3 tablespoons olive oil 1/4 teaspoon pepper

1 teaspoon dried sage leaves

1 tablespoon dried rosemary (if you have fresh, tuck branches and leaves under the string ties)

1 boneless veal shoulder roast, 2 1/2 to 3 pounds, trimmed of fat, rolled and tied

3 cups Chicken stock or broth (substitute for 2 cups stock plus 1 cup dry white wine)

Preheat oven to 350°F. In small bowl mix sage, rosemary, garlic, oil, and pepper. Rub surface of veal with this seasoned oil. Place roast in a large roaster pan with a lid. Pour 2 cups stock around veal. Roast par¬tially covered for 1 hour, turning 2 or 3 times, until barely tender. Uncover and roast until lightly browned, about 15 minutes longer. Remove meat from pan, and tent with foil to keep warm. Put pan juices in a pan over medium heat, and bring juices to a boil, scraping up brown bits from bottom of pan. Add remaining stock to pan. Season with additional pepper to taste. Slice veal roast and serve with pan juices.

From "365 Easy Italian Recipes" by Rick Marzullo O'Connell

LAMB

Armenian Lamb Shanks

8 ripe tomatoes, chopped

1 teaspoon crushed dried oregano

1/2 teaspoon fresh ground black pepper 1/2 teaspoon ground allspice

1/4 teaspoon nutmeg

4 1/2 pounds lamb shanks, sawed in 2-inch pieces 2 medium yellow onions, peeled and sliced

Trim shanks of excess fat, and place in an 8-quart stove-top casserole. Add the remaining ingredients. Bring to a boil and simmer, covered, until the lamb is tender, about 1 1/2 hours. Partially uncover pot for the last 1/2 hour. Garnish with finely chopped yellow onion mixed with parsley.

From: The Frugal Gourmet Jeff Smith

Lamb With Sweet Red Peppers

3 pounds boneless leg of lamb, cut into 1 1/2-inch pieces 1/2 teaspoon pepper

3 tablespoons olive oil 2 garlic cloves, chopped 2 cups hot water

3 tablespoons chopped fresh parsley

2 large red bell peppers, cut into 1 1/2 to 2-inch pieces

Season lamb with 1/4 teaspoon pepper. In a large frying pan or flameproof casserole, heat oil over high heat. Add lamb and cook, turning frequently, 3-5 minutes, or until browned on all sides. Add garlic, water and remaining 1/4 teaspoon pepper. Bring to a boil, reduce heat to medium, and cook partially covered 30 minutes. Uncover and cook 10 minutes longer, or until lamb is fork tender. Add parsley and red peppers to pan. Cook 10 minutes, or until pep¬pers are just tender.

From: "365 Easy Italian Recipes" by Rick Marzullo O'Connell

Rolled Lamb With Garlic

16 garlic cloves, unpeeled

2 tablespoons chopped fresh parsley

2 teaspoons fresh oregano or 3/4 teaspoon dried 1 leg of lamb, boned, 3 1/2 to 4 pounds

3/4 teaspoon pepper

1 1/2 tablespoons olive oil

Preheat oven to 350°F. Bake unpeeled garlic in a small baking pan covered with foil for 15 minutes. Peel garlic. Increase oven tem-perature to 475°F. Set lamb on work surface, boned side up. Scatter whole garlic cloves, parsley, and oregano over lamb. Season with 1/4 teaspoon pepper. Roll up roast and tie at 2-inch intervals. Rub lamb with olive oil. Season with remaining pepper. Place lamb in an open roasting pan. Roast lamb at 475°F. for 15 minutes. Reduce oven temperature to 350°F. and cook 1 hour 15 minutes longer, or until lamb is medium-rare. Serve with pan juices.

From: "365 Easy Italian Recipes" by Rick Marzullo O'Connell

Roast Lamb with Herbs

1 garlic clove, minced

1 teaspoon pepper

1 crushed bay leaf

1/2 teaspoon ginger

1/2 teaspoon marjoram

1/2 teaspoon thyme

1/2 teaspoon sage

1 tablespoon oil

1 leg of lamb

Mix garlic, seasonings, herbs and oil together. Rub on the roast. Place lamb on rack in roasting pan. Cook, uncovered, at 300°F. for approxi¬mately 30 minutes per pound.

From: Mrs. Apoundert N. Zeller, in "Seasoned in Sewickley"

Lamb Chops Stuffed With Chicken Livers

6 chicken livers, chopped

1/2-pound mushrooms, chopped

5 tablespoons olive oil

pepper

1 tablespoon parsley, finely chopped

6 double rib lamb chops

Sauté the livers and mushrooms in 2 tablespoons olive oil, do not let them brown. Season with pepper Add parsley. Trim fat from chops and slit them to make pockets. Stuff with liver mixture. Heat the remain¬ing oil in heavy casserole, add chops and sear them over high heat in both sides. Cover casserole and bake at 350°F. for 25 minutes or until tender. You can skewer chops to close pockets and broil on both sides until cooked. Put chops on a platter, and pour pan juice over them, and serve.

From: Anna Rae Kitay in "Three Rivers Cookbook II"

PORK

Pork Rillettes

1-pound pork fillet

freshly ground black pepper

pinch cayenne pepper

1/4 teaspoon nutmeg 1/2-pound best lard

1/4 pint boiling water

2 bay leaves plus extra for garnish

6 ramekins or small dishes.

Cut pork into 1-inch pieces, place in a bowl and season generous¬ly with freshly ground black pepper. Add cayenne and nutmeg and mix well. Place meat in a heavy based saucepan with the lard and bay leaves. Add water, bring back to the boil then simmer gently for about 45 minutes or until the liquid has reduced by almost half. Remove and toss away bay leaves. Lift out meat with a slotted spoon, strain liquid and keep to one side. Pass the meat through the finest blade of your mincer or put through food processor. Place the minced meat into a bowl and beat in half of the reserved liquid with a wooden spoon. Correct the seasoning and spoon the mixture into ramekins, smoothing over the tops with back of a spoon. Leave to cool. If serving the same day, leave in fridge to cool until ready to serve. If serving later pour over the remaining fat and allow to set over the top of the meat mix. They will keep in fridge this way for up to 2 weeks. To serve, remove the top coating of fat, garnish with bay leaf and serve with celery sticks as a scoop or roll a little in a lettuce leaf and eat with fingers. Serves 6.

From couchman@bigfoot.com

Grilled Pork Chops

1/4 cup fresh lemon juice

2 tablespoons olive oil

3 garlic cloves, minced

1/4 teaspoon ground thyme

1/4 teaspoon dried oregano

1/4 teaspoon black pepper

6 pork chops, 1 inch thick

In a shallow dish, blend all ingredients, except meat. Add pork chops. Cover and chill 12 hours or overnight, turning meat occasionally. To serve, remove meat from marinade. Grill over hot coals 15-20 minutes per side or until done. Baste chops with mari-nade during grilling.

From: Gretchen Hansen in "3 Rivers Cookbook"

Santa Fe Chops With Firecracker Salsa

6 1-1/2-inch-thick boneless pork center loin chops

1 tbsp. chili powder

1 tablespoon ground cumin

1 tablespoon ground black pepper

Mix together seasonings and spread evenly on both surfaces of chops. Place chops on a kettle style grill directly over medium hot coals, lower grill hood and grill for 7-8 minutes; turn chops and grill for 7 minutes more. Serve with Firecracker Salsa on the side.

Firecracker Salsa: In a small bowl, stir together 1 20 ounce can drained pineapple tidbits, 1 medium diced cucumber, 1 tablespoon fresh lime juice, 1 tablespoon honey, and 1 jalapeno chile, seeded and minced. Cover and refrigerate 4-24 hours to let flavors blend.

From: Nat'l Pork Products/Nat'/ Pork Board

Pork Rinds

Buy an untrimmed leg of pig. Slice off the fat layer as thickly as you can, chop to whatever size and shape you prefer, fry in its own fat stirring occasionally to keep the bits apart. Drain as well as you can, sea¬son to taste.

From: rec.food.cooking

SAUSAGE

Deer Sausage

I got this from one of the Frugal Gourmet TV shows- he made it with pork. I've tried it with antelope meat or deer meat. Excellent every time!

Seasonings for

4 pounds ground meat (ground with 2/3 game scraps, 1/3 pork suet)

1 tablespoon fennel seed, freshly ground (I mix all dry spices in the

blender)

3 bay leaves, crushed (it's good with or without this)

3-4 tablespoons minced parsley, fresh or dried

5 cloves fresh garlic minced

1/2 tablespoon red pepper flakes (more or less depending on taste)

3 teaspoons salt

3 tablespoons freshly ground black pepper

Mix all together and refrigerate 24 hours before cooking so that flavors will blend. May use as bulk sausage or, if you happen to have a sausage casing machine, you could make links. We like to use this in spaghetti sauce, or it's great cooked up by itself for a main dish. I also make regular breakfast sausage with deer meat, but I don't have a recipe. I use Morton Sausage Seasoning (salt, sage, coriander and a few other spices). These are good seasonings for any type of meat- with the game meat, remember that it is very lean so you have to add other fat. The flavor is different with beef fat. We like the pork suet for sausage.

From: Julie Jarvis

Breakfast Or Country Sausage

10 pounds pork shoulder

4 tablespoons salt

1 1/2 tablespoons white pepper

2 1/2 tablespoons sage

1 tablespoon nutmeg

1 tablespoon thyme

1 1/2 teaspoons ginger

1/2 tablespoon cayenne pepper

2 cups ice water

Trim the fat off the pork shoulder, if you like lean sausage, or leave it on if you like more flavor. Always make certain that your meat is free of bone and glands. Lumpy likes the 1/8" grinding plate, and recommends grinding the meat only once. To the ground meat, mix in the dry spices first. Then add the ice water. Mix thorough¬ly. Bulk sausage is easily made into patties, or you can use 22- 24mm lamb casings for the challenge of making link sausage. They usually cost between $25.00 - $35.00 per hank (bundle), and can stuff approximately 55 pounds of meat. Wrap the finished product in freezer paper for long term storage, or fry some up right now for a real treat!

From: Panhead. posted to many newsgroups

Texas Hill Country Sausage

4 pounds Pork butt with fat

2 pounds Beef chuck or round - with Fat

1 Large Onion - minced

6 Cloves garlic - minced

2 tablespoons Fresh sage - minced

1 tablespoon Salt

1 tablespoon Fresh ground black pepper

2 tablespoons Crushed red pepper

1 teaspoon Cayenne

4 Yards Hog casings

Coarse grind the meat. Mix in seasonings. Refrigerate overnight. Prepare casings. Stuff to 1" thick, 5" long and tie off. They can be frozen or refrigerated at this time. To smoke: rub sausages with oil. Don't overdo it or they get messy and then turn to mush. Smoke at 225°F..for two hours with oak or mesquite until the skin looks ready to pop.

Recipe By: Smoke and Spice; From: "Garry Howard" <garhow@tiac.Nef>; MM by Helen Peagram. Posted to rec. food. preserving; Recipe via Meal-Master

Texas Smoky Links

2 pounds Pork butt

1-pound Beef chuck

1 teaspoon Ground coriander

2 teaspoons Ground cumin

2 teaspoons Chopped garlic

1 tablespoon Ground black pepper

2 teaspoons Red pepper flakes

1/2 cup Ice water

4 teaspoons Salt

pinch of Ground allspice

pinch of Ground cloves

Grind pork 3/8 plate-beef 1/4" plate- mix and stuff in hog casings - 8" links. Hot smoke to 155°F. or cold smoke at least 12 hours.

Recipe By: John "Smoky" Mitchell; From: "Garry Howard" <garhow@tiac.Nef>; MM by Helen Peagram. Posted to rec.food.preserving

BAKED CHICKEN

Italian Chicken

2 tablespoons olive oil

2 tablespoons lemon juice

1 clove garlic, crushed

1/4 teaspoon dried oregano

1/8 teaspoon pepper

Mix all in a shallow dish. Add 4 pieces of chicken, turning to coat well. Cover and refrigerate for 8-12 hours, remember to turn it over occasionally. One hour before serving, heat oven to 450°F. Line a baking

sheet with foil, and put chicken on. Put pan in oven, reduce heat to 325°F. Bake 35-45minutes.

From JoAnn <jdynbttn@sgi.net>

Mandarin Chicken Salad

2scallions, sliced

6 tablespoons olive oil

1/4teaspoon pepper

1/2cup coarsely chopped pecans

2 cups diced (1/2inch) cooked chicken

1 bunch watercress, tough stems removed

111-ounce can mandarin oranges, rinsed well, drained and chilled

2 tablespoons lemon or lime juice (substitute for red wine vinegar)

Preheat oven to 325°F. Spread out pecans on a small baking sheet Bake for 10-15minutes, until lightly toasted. In a salad bowl, combine chicken, watercress, oranges, scallions and toasted pecans. Drizzle on oil, juice, and pepper. Toss to coat.

Adapted from "365 Ways to Cook Chicken" by Cheryl Sedaker.

Garlic Chicken

1/4cup olive oil

1 large onion, diced pepper to taste

juice of 2 lemons

2 large carrots, sliced

4 celery stalks, sliced

23-pound chickens, cut into pieces, no backs or wings

20-30 garlic cloves, unpeeled and left whole (that's right, "twenty to thirty"!)

Heat the oil in a frying pan. Add the onion, carrots and celery, stirring constantly, until they are soft. With a slotted spoon, transfer the vegetables to a casserole dish with a tight-fitting lid, or to a clay pot. lay the chicken pieces on top of the vegetables. Sprinkle with pepper and lemon juice. Put the garlic around and on the chicken pieces. Cover tightly, this is essential, because the chicken must cook in its own juices. Cook in a preheated 350°F. oven for 1 hour. Do not uncover until ready to serve.

From "Nika Haze/ton's Way with Vegetables"

Macadamia Nut Chicken

Take some chicken breasts, pound thin. Coat with pesto (sans parmesan), then coat with crushed macadamias. Bake about 1/2 hour at around 350 or so.

From JoAnn <jdynbttn@sgi.net>

Chicken Cutlets with Olives and Tomatoes

Large foil pan or two 9x13 pans, greased or lightly sprayed

6 skinless chicken breasts

6 cloves garlic, chopped

1 large onion, chopped

3 tablespoons extra virgin olive oil

juice of 1 lemon

16 ounce can plum tomatoes, drained and chopped or equivalent amount of fresh plum tomatoes, blanched to remove skin and chopped

18 black olives, drained, pitted and chopped (about 1/2 can)

3 tablespoons fresh parsley, chopped fine (divided)

2 teaspoons fresh thyme (chopped)

salt and freshly ground pepper to taste

375°F. oven. Marinate chicken in 2 tablespoons oil, lemon juice and salt and pepper for one hour, turning often. In a large skillet sauté garlic and onions in remaining 1 tablespoon olive oil. Add tomatoes and olives and sauté for 15 minutes, uncovered, stirring often. Add 1 tablespoon of the parsley and all of the thyme, stirring to combine. Place the chicken breasts in the prepared pans and cover with sauteed mixture. Sprinkle with remaining parsley. Bake for 35 - 40 minutes in a 375°F. oven or until brown. Yield: 8 - 10 main course portions

From: MS Dietary Home Page http://www.2x2.eo.nz/msl

CROCK POT CHICKEN

Chicken In-A-Pot

3-pound whole chicken

2 carrots, sliced

2 onions, sliced

2 celery stalks with leaves, cut in 1-inch pieces

1 teaspoon basil

1/2 teaspoon salt

1/2 teaspoon black pepper

1/2 cup chicken broth

Put carrots, onions, and celery in bottom of crock-pot. Add whole chicken. Top with salt, pepper, liquid. Sprinkle basil over top. Cover and cook until done-low 8 to 10 hours. (High 3 to 4 hours, using 1 cup water). Remove chicken and vegetables with spatula. Yield: 6 servings

From: rec.food.recipes archives

Chicken Veggie Packets

4 boneless skinless chicken breast halves, about 1-pound 1/2-pound fresh mushrooms, sliced

1 1/2 cups baby carrots, halved lengthwise 1 cup frozen pearl onions, thawed

1/2 cup julienned sweet red pepper 1/4 teaspoon pepper

1 teaspoon dried thyme

Flatten chicken breasts to 1/2-inch thickness; place each on a piece of heavy-duty foil, about 12"xl2". Layer mushrooms, car¬rots, onions and red pepper over chicken, sprinkle with thyme and pepper. Fold foil around chicken and vegetables and seal tightly. Place on a baking sheet. Bake at 375°F. for 20 minutes, or until chicken juices run clear. Makes 4 servings.

From: Edna Shaffer in Quick Cooking, JIF '99

Chicken Curry With Apple

2 tablespoons olive oil

1 cup chopped onion

1 cup chopped peeled apple

1 can (16 ounce) stewed tomatoes with their own juice

1 cup chicken broth

1 teaspoon lemon juice

1 tablespoon curry powder or more to taste

4 cups chopped cooked chicken

garnishes: toasted coconut, mandarin oranges, raisins, crumbled cooked bacon, mango chutney, chopped onion

Heat oil in a large frying pan over medium heat. Add onion and cook until softened, about 3 minutes. Add apple, tomatoes and their juice, broth, lemon juice, and curry powder. Simmer, uncovered, 35 minutes. Add chicken and heat through, about 5 minutes. Serve with assorted garnishes on the side.

From "365 Ways to Cook Chicken" by Cheryl Sedaker

Chicken Vindaloo

Introduced to India by Portuguese settlers, this spicy stew can also be made with pork, beef or lamb.

1/3 cup lime or lemon juice 6 large garlic cloves, peeled

3 tablespoons chopped fresh ginger 1 1/2 tablespoons curry powder

2 teaspoons ground cumin

3/4 teaspoon ground cardamom 1/4 teaspoon ground cloves

1/4 teaspoon (generous) dried crushed red pepper 2 tablespoons yellow mustard seed

2 pounds skinless boneless chicken thighs (about 10), cut into 1-to 1 1/2-inch pieces

4 tablespoons olive oil

2 1/2 cups chopped onions

1 14 1/2- to 16-ounce can diced tomatoes in juice 1 cinnamon stick

1/2 cup chopped fresh cilantro

Place first 8 ingredients in blender. Add 1 tablespoon mustard seeds and blend until smooth. Transfer spice mixture to large bowl. Add chicken and 2 tablespoons oil and toss to coat well. Heat remaining 2 tablespoons oil in heavy large pot over medium-high heat. Add onions and sauté until golden, about 5 minutes. Add chicken mixture and stir 3 minutes to blend flavors. Add tomatoes with their juice and cinna¬mon stick; bring to boil. Reduce heat; cover and simmer until chicken is tender, stirring occasionally, about 30 minutes. Season chicken mix¬ture to taste with salt and pepper. Mix in remaining 1 tablespoon mus¬tard seeds. Simmer uncovered until liquid is slightly thickened, about 8 minutes. Remove cinnamon stick. Stir in cilantro and serve. Makes 4 Servings

Courtesy ofwww.mustardstore.com

Grilled Jamaican Jerk Chicken

15 of your favorite fresh chile peppers (or equivalent)

2 tablespoons dried rosemary

2 tablespoons parsley, chopped

2 tablespoons dried basil

2 tablespoons dried thyme

2 tablespoons mustard seeds

3 scallions, finely chopped

1 teaspoon salt

1 teaspoon black pepper

juice of 2 limes

1/4 cup cheap yellow mustard

2 tablespoons orange juice

6 chicken thighs, with legs attached

Combine all the rub ingredients in a food processor, or blender, and blend them into a paste, making sure that all the ingredients are fully integrated. The paste should be approximately the con-sistency of a thick tomato sauce. If it is too thick, thin it out with a little more white vinegar. Cover the paste and let it sit in the refrig¬erator for at least 2 hours for the flavors to blend together. Overnight is the ideal amount of time to give them to get acquainted. (*NOTE If you want to avoid making a fresh batch every time you make this dish, you can multiply the amount of paste easily. Don't worry about it going bad, since it keeps almost infinitely.) Rub the chicken thighs with paste and place them on the grill over very low heat. If you have a covered cooker, put the coals to one side and the chicken on the other, and cover. Cook about 1 hour without a cover or 1/2 hour if covered. The key here is to use a very low heat. You need to be patient and give yourself plenty of time. The chicken is technically done when the meat is opaque and the juices run clear. However, the ideal is about 10-15 minutes past that point, when the meat pulls away from the bone easily. It is very hard to overcook this. In fact, you can only screw it up if you burn the paste by having the heat too high. The longer the chicken stays on the grill, the more superior the smoky flavor. After cooking, separate the leg from the thigh by cutting at the natural joint between them. Serve one leg or thigh per person accompanied by a few spoonful's of Banana-guava ketchup. Serves 4 and as entree or 6 as a light meal.

Origin: Cookbook Digest magazine, July/Aug 1991

GRILLED AND BROILED CHICKEN

Grilled Picante Chicken

4 boneless, skinless chicken breasts

1 cup picante sauce

Marinate chicken in picante sauce for about 5 hours in the refrigera¬tor (or longer if desired). Place on grill when hot enough. Brush mari¬nade on chicken, turn after five minutes and brush marinade on other side. Do not use the marinade after the first few minutes, because the marinade could contain raw chicken juices. Chicken takes about 15 minutes to cook, until no longer pink inside.

From Pam at http:llwww.ilovejesus.com/lot/locarb/

Lemon Chicken Kebabs

1/4 cup olive oil

2 tablespoons fresh lemon juice 3 garlic cloves, crushed

1/2 teaspoon coarsely cracked pepper

1 1/4-pound skinless, boneless chicken breasts, cut into bite sized pieces

Preheat broiler, or light your grill. Soak wooden skewers in water for 20 minutes to prevent them burning. Meanwhile, in a small bowl, combine oil, lemon juice, garlic and pepper. Add chicken pieces, and toss to coat. Marinate 15 minutes. Thread 3 or 4 chicken pieces onto each wooden skewer, reserve marinade. Grill chicken over hot coals, baste frequently with marinade and turning, for 12-15 minutes. Or broil, turn frequently, for about 5 minutes.

From "365 Ways to Cook Chicken" by Cheryl Sedaker.

Spice-Crusted Chicken Breast

1 tablespoon ground coriander

1 tablespoon ground cumin

1 teaspoon freshly ground black pepper

4 boned and skinned chicken breast halves

2 teaspoons olive oil

In a small dry skillet, over medium heat, toast coriander, cumin and pepper, stirring, for 45 seconds or until aromatic. Transfer to a small bowl and set aside. Preheat broiler. Lightly oil a broiler rack or coat it with cooking spray. Place chicken breasts between two pieces of plastic wrap; flatten the meat slightly with a rolling pin. Brush both sides of the chicken with oil, then coat with spice mixture and place on broiler rack. Broil until the chicken is no longer pink in the center, four to five minutes per side. per serv¬ing: 3 lean meat, 1/2 fat. 127 calories, 3.9 g fat, 1.7 g carbohydrate, 593 mg sodium.

Bacon-Y Chicken Thighs

2 pounds chicken thighs 1/4-pound bacon

1 cup chicken broth

Cut bacon into 1" pieces. Cook in iron skillet until done. Remove bacon to drain. In same skillet over medium heat, cook the chick¬en in the bacon fat until brown on all sides, about 10 minutes. Spoon out the bacon grease. Pour in the broth, heat to boil, reduce heat to low, cover and simmer 20-30 minutes, until chick¬en is fork tender. Throw bacon back in, and you're done.

From: JoAnn <jdynbttn@sgi.net>

Chicken A La Nancy

4 skinless boneless chicken breast halves

1/4 cup olive oil

1 garlic clove, finely chopped

1/2-pound mushrooms, sliced

1/2 lemon, thinly sliced

1/4 teaspoon pepper

1/4 teaspoon oregano

1/2 cup chicken broth (substituted for dry white wine)

1 tablespoon arrowroot powder (substituted for flour)

1 14 ounce can whole artichoke hearts, drained and quartered

Pound chicken breasts to 1/4" thickness between sheets of plastic wrap or wax paper. Cut into 2-inch squares. In a large fry pan, heat oil over medium heat. Add chicken and cook 2-3 minutes a side, until tender and opaque. Remove chicken and keep warm. Add garlic, lemon and mushrooms to the same pan. Cook until tender, 3-5 minutes. Sprinkle with arrowroot powder, pepper and oregano. Cook, stirring, 1 minute. Add broth, and bring to a boil, stirring until mixture thickens. Add artichokes and return chicken to pan. Simmer 2 minutes, until heated through.

From: Frank Perdue in "365 Ways to Cook Chicken"

"Breaded" Chicken Strips

I made some chicken strips that I breaded with dried onions and sesame seeds. Just dip chicken (or whatever) in egg, then roll in a mix¬ture of equal parts dried onion and sesame seeds. I fried them in olive oil, but I'm sure you could use side pork drippings. You can grind up the dried onions to make a flour and forget the sesame seeds if you did¬n't want it so crispy.

From: Patti Vincent

GAME BIRDS

Grilled Quail Salad With

Provencal Vegetables and Lime Dressing

4 boned quail [or you could prepare with the bone in]

1 cup Lime Dressing [recipe in Salad Dressings]

Separate the quail legs from the breasts and arrange the pieces in a single layer in a bowl with the Lime Dressing. Marinate in the refrig¬erator the quail for 8-12 hours. Grill or broil the quail until medium rare. Slice each breast crosswise into pieces. Makes appetizer-size serv¬ings

From: "French Food American Accent" by Debra Ponzek

Deep Fried Quail

birds

8 cloves garlic

2 centers lemon grass

1 tablespoon black pepper (crushed)

1/4 cup olive oil

This is rather low-rent, but my favorite quail dish is deep-fried. Take your birds and marinate them with garlic, lemon grass, black pepper (crushed) and oil overnight. Reduce marinade to a fine emulsion in a mortar and rub it into the quail (inside the body cavity, under the skins, etc.)

Allow them to come to room temperature, dry them off, and then deep fry them in oil. They'll puff up and then deflate. Cook them to your taste (either very crispy or not so). I serve them Vietnamese-style with salt and pepper powder (roast white pep-percorns with salt and some lemon zest, then crush) and limes. Squeeze the lime on the quail, dip in salt/pepper combo, and eat. They are great served with pickled carrots and daikon (again, Vietnamese-style). Your numbers may be slightly off. I would allow 3-4 quail per person (I tend to get very small birds). They are quite addictive served this way and you'll be surprised how many you end up eating (bones and all!)

From: lapageria@aol.com in RFC

WILD GAME

Here are some good preparation tips:

http://www.exoticmeats.com/Web_store/web_store.cgi?page=CookingEM.html

Alligator Etouffee

1-pound alligator meat (cut in thin strips)

1 cup olive oil

1/2 cup green onions (chopped)

1/4 cup parsley (chopped)

2 garlic cloves (minced)

4 celery stalks (chopped)

1 can tomatoes (sorry, no size given)

salt, cayenne and black pepper

Sauté onions, garlic and celery in butter until soft. Add tomatoes and simmer for 20 minutes in covered iron pot. Add alligator meat and allow to cook over low heat until tender (approximately 1 hour). If gravy is too thick, add a little hot water.

September, 1990 - Louisiana Conservationist Calendar: Posted by Fred Towner

<fownerf@cyberlink.bc.ca> to rec.food.recipes

Bear Roast

4 pounds Bear meat

Pepper to taste

Celery salt to taste

2 Garlic cloves

8-ounce (piece) Salt pork

Season the bear meat with the celery salt and pepper and place in a stock pot, adding the garlic, salt pork, and enough water to cover; Cook until meat is tender, then drain RESERVING the pan juices. Place the meat in a roasting pan and top with the onions, roast at 350°F. until brown, basting with the reserved juices. Thicken the remaining juices for gravy. Yield: 12 servings

From: Fred Towner <townerf@cyberlink.bc.ca> in rec.food.recipes archives: Adapted by Patti Vincent

Elk Tenderloin With Brandy Mustard Sauce

2 elk tenderloins,

8-10 ounce each sliced bacon

1/2 cup sliced mushrooms

1 tablespoon Grey Poupon mustard

1/4 cup onion, finely diced

1/4 cup bell pepper, diced

1/2 cup brown gravy

1 clove garlic

thyme

ground black pepper

Remove silver skin from tenderloins and rub meat with split garlic cloves. Sprinkle lightly with thyme and black pepper. Wrap bacon around tenderloin and use toothpick to secure. Place in hot frying pan and sauté until bacon is cooked. Note: tenderloins should not be cooked past medium rare. Remove from pan and pour off excess grease. Place onion and bell pepper in pan for 30 seconds, add mushrooms and sauté until tender.

Adapted from Bill Parton, Chef, Buckhorn Exchange Restaurant

Grilled Rattlesnake With Mojo Criollo

It's so strange that I actually have some rattlesnake recipes! We actu¬ally cooked up a rattler at a friend's house (he lives way out in the Mojave Desert of California and has tons of those things crawling around his yard). After cutting off its head and skinning and gutting it, we marinated the snake in Mojo Criollo, a Cuban marinating sauce consisting of lots of garlic and sour orange juice. We allowed it to mar¬inate for a couple of hours, then we grilled it. Muy delicioso! I usually buy bottled Mojo in the store, but in the Marinade section is a recipe that's pretty close to the bottled version.

From: Stace Hiatt in rec.food.recipes

Rattlesnake

We usually add rattlesnake to chili. Treat rattlesnake as you would any quick-cooking white meat (i.e., chicken, shellfish). Of course, everyone will tell you it "tastes just like chicken". It is also very good deep fried in a simple "breading." You might try looking for fried alligator recipes too and adapt them for use with your snake. If your rattler is still alive or in one piece, the following directions for dressing rattlesnakes might be helpful:

1. Place dead rattlesnake on a cutting board and hold firmly behind the head.

2. Cut off head and rattles and discard.

3. Strip of skin and discard or save (for a hat band maybe?)

4. Make along slice along the underside and remove all internal organs.

5. Cut into chunks and refrigerate or freeze until ready to use.

From: l Hodge in rec.food.cooking

Barbecued Venison Steaks With Herbs

4 Venison Steaks (4 ounce each)

Chopped rosemary

2 Tablespoon Chopped garlic

2 Tablespoon Chopped thyme

2 Tablespoon Olive oil 1/4 cup

pepper to taste

For marinade, combine oil and herbs. Marinate venison for 4 hours in refrigerator, covered. Remove from marinade and shake off excess oil. Place venison on grill over just hot coals (but not flaming). Season with pepper and brush with marinade. Cook for 5 minutes turning once, or until medium rare.

From http://www.foodcomm.com/recipes/

Roasted Venison The Easy Way

Venison Roast, about 1 1/2 pounds

Olive oil, enough to coat meat

Heat roasting pan until hot. Add olive oil to coat and brown veni-son on each side. Cook in oven at 375°F. for 15-20 minutes or until medium rare. Let it stand for 5 minutes and carve into thin (1/2-inch-thick) slices. Suggested Accompaniments: Sauteed leeks with wild mushrooms.

From http://www.foodcomm.comkecipes/index.htm

Grilled Venison Brochettes

Venison Leg or Shoulder Roast, 2 pounds

4 Baby artichokes, halved

2 Bell peppers (any color)

3/4 cup Olive oil

3 tablespoons Chopped fresh basil

2 tablespoons Lemon juice

1 tablespoon Red chili flakes

Pepper to taste

For marinade, combine olive oil, basil, lemon juice and chili flakes. Roast and peel peppers. Cut into 2-inch squares. For venison, cut veni¬son roast in 1-1/2-inch cubes. Marinate venison and vegetables for 30 minutes. Thread skewer with venison and vegetables. Grill over high heat for 5-6 minutes, turning once. Venison should be rare. Brush with marinade just before serving.

From http:llwww.foodcomm.com/recipes/

Italian-Style Venison Pot Roast

3-4 pounds venison pot roast

2 tablespoons fat

pepper

1 8 ounce can tomato sauce

1 medium onion, chopped

1 cup celery, chopped

1 Tablespoon. parsley, minced

2 teaspoon oregano

1 clove garlic

1 cup dry red wine (I know wine isn't Diet Evolution compliant- come up with a substitute)

In Dutch oven, brown roast on all sides in fat. Add pepper to taste. Combine remaining ingredients, and pour over pot roast. Cover and bake 3 to 4 hours at 300°F.

Adapted from Theresa J. Famey, Colorado Springs Sun

Venison Grilled Tenderloins

Wash and trim the tenderloins well. Rub with white pepper and garlic. Make a sauce of Ray's Neanderthin barbeque sauce, honey and lemon pepper seasoning and marinate the tenderloins. Roll the tenderloin up in foil and place it on the back of the grill. Cook slowly at low flame.

From Vance Persall

Roast Loin of Venison

4 pounds boneless loin of venison, at room temperature

2 tablespoons olive oil

1 teaspoon freshly ground pepper

1/2 teaspoon finely chopped juniper berries

Preheat the oven to 400°F. Rub the venison with the olive oil, 1 teaspoon of the pepper and 1/2 teaspoons of the chopped juniper berries, pressing the seasonings into the meat. Set the loin on a rack in a roasting pan and roast, basting frequently with the pan juices, until medium-rare (about 135°F. on a meat thermometer), 25 to 30 minutes. Cover the venison loosely with foil and set aside for 10 to 15 minutes before carving. Slice the venison thinly.

Adapted from http:!lwww.mcs.vuw.ac.nz/school/staff/Amy-Gale.html

Venison Roasted In A Pinenut Crust

Venison hind leg

1/2 cup ground pinenuts

1 teaspoon crushed garlic

1 teaspoon coarse black pepper

6 pitted figs (optional)

6 dried apricots (optional)

3 diced ginger (optional)

1/2 teaspoon ground allspice (optional)

5 crushed juniper berries (optional)

Combine crust ingredients and press onto top and side of meat. Transfer meat to a roasting dish and roast at 220°C for about 12 minutes allowing minutes per centimeter depth of meat. Rest meat for 8-10 minutes before carving. Optional - The meat can be stuffed with the fruit mixture before coating with the crust. Carefully cut a pocket lengthwise in the venison using a long narrow knife taking care not to pierce the outer flesh. Dice dried fruits finely and combine with ginger, allspice, juniper berries and brandy. Fill cavity of meat with fruit mixture and secure cavity hole with toothpicks. To cook by microwave - This is best done without a nut coating. Stuff the meat. Brown well in a lightly oiled pan. Transfer the meat to a plate and cover loosely with a paper towel. Microwave at full power for 2 -3 minutes. Leave to stand for 8 minutes before slicing.

From http:/www.foodcomm.com/recipes/

Venison Chili

About 2 pounds of venison or venison burger (cube the venison into small chunks about 1/2 inch to 1-inch square; if there are any bones, save to use in the chili to enrich the sauce)

2 large onions, sliced

10 cloves of garlic, finely minced

1 quart of chicken stock, preferably homemade without salt

4 tablespoons of chili powder (use plain chili powder, without any salt or other spices in it - you may purchase this at a health food store with bins for spices)

1 tablespoon ground cumin

2 tablespoons sweet red paprika

1 teaspoon of cayenne pepper

Palmful of dried oregano (this is a couple of tablespoons or so) ground between your hands

3 bay leaves

1 teaspoon of kosher salt

1/4 cup olive oil [was other oil]

Brown the venison in batches until brown on all sides. Remove to a dish. When all the venison is browned, sauté the onions in the remain¬ing oil. You want the onions to melt but not brown. When the onions have reached the melt stage (about 10 minutes) add the garlic. Don't let the garlic burn. Just let it scent up. Add the browned meat, the stock, the chili powder, cumin, cayenne, paprika, bay leaves, oregano, salt and stock. Bring to a boil. Reduce heat to a just barely simmering and cover. Simmer gently covered for 3 hours. The meat should be fork tender. Even though venison is very lean, the chili should be defatted. I do this by letting it cool and then refrigerating the chili overnight. The next day, I remove the fat. To serve, reheat. Taste for seasoning. Sometimes, I add a bit more cumin. Some like to thicken the chili with masa or fine corn meal. To do this, mix some about 1/4 cup fine corn meal with enough water to make a thin paste (no more than one cup of water). Add this quickly to the chili as it simmers, stir like crazy, or you may get lumps. If you use the masa, be sure to cook the chili for at least another 20 minutes or so, or it may taste pasty. Coleslaw would be the only salad I'd serve with this. If there's any chili left, and this should feed six adults, it freezes beautifully. Enjoy!

Note: This makes a sprightly but not firey chile. If you want to go for the burn, use hamburger or top round and add several jalapeno peppers, seeds and all. No point wasting good venison on fire, so use beef or pork.

ORGAN MEATS

All organ meats should be really fresh. You want to take them home and ideally cook them the same day your butcher puts them out. Sweetbreads take a bit of preparation time. It can be either calf thymus, (calf's sweetbreads), or beef pancreas. I suppose it could also be calf pancreas, too. Soak them in really cold water, changing every 20 min or so, for an hour. Then peel whatever you can of the capsule surrounding the sweetbreads.

Next simmer them for about 20 min, in water with a little lemon juice, and a bay leaf if you like. Remove, rinse in cold water, remove any more membrane (but don't get too obsessive about this), and they are ready to use in any recipe you might like. My favorite is slice about the width of a finger (use a sharp knife), and sauté gently with olive oil, mushrooms, and a few chopped shallots.

They are also good sliced and broiled, say brushed with olive oil. Maybe 8 to 10 minutes per side, about 6" from the heat. Lemon juice squeezed over them at serving hits the spot.

They can be baked, too. Almost anything after the initial cleaning and simmering. Kidneys are different, here the problem is controlling the production of an ammonia smell, that pretty well kills the appetite. Best are calf's or lamb's kidneys, and most of ours in the past have been lamb, that a local woman would give me for helping her butcher them. With these, if they smell really good, I just trim off the fat and white gristle, slice 1/2" or so thick, or cube, and grill over charcoal. (The cube on a skewer with onion, green pepper, and tomato.) The secret here is really hot, and not too long. If the calf is closer to a beef, or the lamb a sheep, slice and soak for a couple of hours in milk (in the fridge), pat dry, then grill or fry in hot olive oil for a short time. The difficulty is that water may start to cook out, and they can get tough. This is usually a sign that the oil wasn't hot enough. Also, any marinade that you like (and fits your diet can be used). The milk is more of a pre-treatment.

From Michael <.mrbuji@WHIDBEY.NET>

Beef And Chicken Liver

I'm trying to use more organ meats for my family. The easiest and most available is beef liver, and chicken livers. Most recipes call for breading them, but I have had delicious results from marinating in oil and lemon juice. Then sauté them in a fair amount of olive oil, HOT, for a short while. Beef liver about 3/8" thick is done in 2 minutes per side. The chicken livers I divide in two before cooking. Then sauté some onions, and combine the meat with the onions just before serv¬ing. Beef heart is good too, and especially good as a shish kebob ingredient. I also fix kidney and sweetbreads (pancreas), but they are more trouble, and also harder to find in the supermar-ket. Sweetbreads are so good, that some of my kids have requested them as a birthday din¬ner!

From Michael <mrbuji@WHJDBEY.NET>

Beef Heart

Made this last night and thought it was swell. Had been cooking some beef heart in bacon grease. Put one large, wedged, not peeled apple in leftover hot grease. Juice of one lemon, about 2 tablespoons raisins, 2 tablespoons chopped walnuts and some cinnamon. Cooked, tossing, until softish. Very good for side dish/dessert.

From Beverly Sweitzer <11bemco@COMM-PLUS.NET>

Beef Tongue with Spicy Sauce

1 Fresh beef tongue

2 Onions

1 large Carrot

4 Sprigs parsley

1 Stalk celery

1/2 Bay leaf

8 Peppercorns

2 teaspoons Salt

Scrub tongue and place in large kettle with onions, carrot, parsley, celery, bay leaf, peppercorns and salt. Cover with boiling water, bring to boil. Skim and simmer, covered, for 3 to 4 hours or until tender. Reserve the tongue liquid in case some is needed for the sauce. Remove the skin and root ends. Strain following sauce over tongue when ready to serve. Serves eight.

Spicy Sauce

1/8 teaspoon ginger

1/2 cup Raw cranberries

1 tablespoon raw honey

1/2 Lemon, sliced and quartered

Combine ginger, cranberries, honey and lemon. Add enough water to cover cranberries. Simmer about 15 minutes. Mash cranberries, and lemon. Check seasoning. If more liquid is needed, use tongue liquor.

Source: "The Best of Shaker Cooking; Revised and Expanded" by Amy Bess. Adapted by Patti Vincent

Tongue

1 3-pound large beef tongue

1 Onion, quartered

1 Carrot, sliced

3 Ribs of leafy celery

6 Sprigs of parsley

2 Bay leaves

10 Peppercorns, cracked

1 Dried chile, optional

All are tasty. They can be purchased fresh, smoked and pickled. The most desired, in order of preference, are: calf, lamb, beef and pork. To prepare: scrub the tongue well. If it is smoked or pickled you may wish to blanch it first, by simmering for about 10 min¬utes. Immerse the tongue in seasoned boiling water to cover, reduce heat and simmer gently for at least one hour. Up to 3 hours for large beef tongues. Then drain, plunge into cold water to cool the meat enough to handle, skin it, and trim any bones and gris¬tle from the root. Finally return it to the cooking water to re-heat it before serving. Or chill it entirely and serve as a cold-cut. To carve, start by cutting through the hump parallel to the base, but towards the tip cut on the diagonal for a better looking presentation. Yields 9 servings

Basque Tongue Stew

1 3-1/2 pound fresh beef tongue

2 carrots, chopped

1/2 bunch parsley

2 bay leaves

10 black peppercorns

1 medium yellow onion, peeled and quartered

1 recipe Basque Tomato Sauce (see Vegetable recipe section for this one)

In a 6-quart pot, place tongue, onion, carrots, parsley, bay leaves, and peppercorns. Add just enough water to cover. Simmer, covered for 2 1/2 hours. Remove tongue, cool, peel, and slice 1/4-inch thick cross¬wise. Add to prepared sauce. Simmer, covered, for 1 hour. Then uncov¬er the pot, and simmer gently 1 1/2 hours, stirring occasionally.

From The Frugal Gourmet Jeff Smith

FISH

Ku Poke, Or Raw Fish With Seaweed

1-pound raw fish, tuna or salmon, cubed, skinless, boneless

1 cup seaweed (hijiki in Japanese markets) The seaweed will be dried, so soak it for 30 minutes in warm water. Then drain and rinse well.

1 small red chile pepper, seeded and chopped

Mix all of the ingredients, and allow the dish to chill a few hours before serving.

From: The Frugal Gourmet Jeff Smith

Lomi-Lomi Salmon

1-pound fresh salmon fillet juice of 1 lemon

2 green onions or 1 sweet yellow onion

lettuce leaves, for dipping

1-pound ripe tomatoes, peeled, seeded and chopped

Place salmon in a large glass or ceramic bowl. Sprinkle salmon with lemon juice. Cover and marinate in refrigerator overnight. Drain salmon. Cover with cold water, and soak 2 hours, changing water 2 or 3 times. Drain well. Pull salmon meat away from bones and skin by hand, discard skin and bones. Massage salmon with fingertips until thoroughly mashed. Add tomatoes and green onions and continue massaging until mixture is smooth. Chill 3 minutes before serving. Serve with lettuce leaves. Serves 6-8.

From: "Regional American Classics'; California Culinary Academy.

Tunisian Spiced Fish

1/2 teaspoon cumin seeds

1/2 teaspoon coriander seeds

1/2 teaspoon dried hot pepper flakes

1/2 teaspoon caraway seeds

1 1/2 pounds cod fillets (snapper or bluefish will do)

3 cloves garlic, thinly sliced

1 medium onion, thinly sliced

parsley for garnish

1 cup fish stock or bottled clam juice

Heat a skillet over medium heat. Add seeds and flakes. Roast for 2- 3 minutes until fragrant. Grind spices in a spice grinder [I used a mortar and pestle and it worked ok). Spread spices on fish. Let stand 10 minutes. Spray an ovenproof dish large enough to fit all the fish in one layer. Add 1/2 garlic, onions and tomato. Add fish. Add remaining garlic, and onions. Pour over fish stock/clam juice over fish. Bake in a preheated 400°F. for 20-30 minutes, depend¬ing on the thickness of the fillets.

From: http://lark.cc.ukans.edu/~lash/recipes!

Basque Codfish Pil Pil

1-pound salt cod, skinless and boneless

3 tablespoons olive oil

4 cloves garlic, peeled and crushed

pinch of red pepper flakes

1 cup chicken stock, simmered with a 1-inch piece of lemon peel

1 egg, beaten

Cut the salt cod into 1-inch wide serving pieces and rinse well. Soak for 24 hours or more, rinsing with fresh water several times. Cook the salt cod in fresh water for about 15 minutes, or until it can be easily flaked, but leave the pieces whole. Drain and let cool, discarding the liquid. Heat a large frying pan and add the oil and crushed garlic. Sauté over medium heat until the garlic barely begins to brown. Add the red pepper flakes, the drained cod, and the chicken stock. Bring to a simmer while shaking the pan gently. With a pancake turner, remove cod to a platter. Turn off the heat, add the beaten egg, and return to low heat. Stir the liquid constantly until the sauce begins to thicken. Remove from heat, and immediately pour over fish and serve.

From: The Frugal Gourmet Jeff Smith

Italian-Style Baccala

1-pound Baccala (dried salted codfish)

1 tablespoon extra-virgin olive oil

3 or 4 cloves garlic, finely minced

1 red onion, cut lengthwise into thin slices

1 red bell pepper, roasted over a flame, peeled, seeded and cut into thin strips

2-3 tsp. capers, drained and lightly rinsed

10-12 oil-cured ripe olives, pitted and coarsely minced

parsley sprigs and lemon wedges for garnish

Soak the Baccala for 48 hours, changing the water every 8 hours to remove the excess salt from the curing process. Heat oil in a deep skil¬let over medium heat. Add garlic and onion and sauté for 2-3 minutes. Add bell pepper, capers and olives and cook for 2-3 minutes. Spread vegetables evenly over bottom of the skillet. Cut Baccala into 4 equal portions. Place on top of the vegetables and add about 1/8 inch of water. Cover and steam over medium heat about 10 minutes, until Baccala is tender and flakes easily. and liquid has evaporated. Gently transfer fish to a serving platter and top with cooked vegetables. Serve immediately, garnished with parsley and lemon wedges. Makes 4 servings.

From: "Cooking the Whole Foods Way" by Christina Pirello.

Thai Salmon Steaks In Panang Curry Sauce

2 8-ounce salmon steaks

2 teaspoons Thai Panang curry base (don't know if this is DE)

1/2 cup chicken broth

4 teaspoons white wine

1/2 cup coconut milk

In a saucepan dissolve the curry base in the chicken stock. Bring to a boil. Add the white wine and simmer for several minutes. Stir in coconut milk; return to a boil. Simmer for several minutes. Sauce will thicken slightly. Serve sauce over broiled salmon steaks.

Snapper Ceviche

1-pound red snapper fillets

7 limes, juiced

2 medium tomatoes

4 serrano chiles

1/4 cup olive oil

1/2 teaspoon salt, or to taste

1/2 teaspoon oregano pepper, to taste

1 small avocado, sliced

1 small onion, sliced into rings

cilantro, minced

Cut the fish into small cubes, about 1/2 inch, and cover them with the lime juice. Set the fish aside in the bottom of refrigerator for at least five hours or until the fish loses its transparent look and becomes opaque. Stir the pieces from time to time so they get evenly cooked in the juice. Skin, seed and chop the tomatoes; chop the chiles with their seeds, and add them with the rest of the ingredients to the fish. Set the ceviche aside in the bottom of the refrigerator for at least 1 hour to season. Serve it chilled, but not so cold that the oil congeals. Before serving, garnish each portion with slices of avocado and onion rings and sprinkle with a little cilantro. Yield: 6 Servings

From: Mr. Bill in rec.food.cooking

Walnut Stuffed Trout

6 fresh trout, boned

2 tablespoons olive oil (substitute for 1/4 cup butter)

1 cup walnuts

2 shallots

1/2 bunch parsley

1/2 teaspoon pepper

1/4 cup olive oil (substitute for 1/2 cup butter)

lemon, parsley, and seedless grapes for garnish

Rinse and dry the trout. Make stuffing: chop walnuts in a food processor until they are fine (save 6 walnuts for garnish). Remove. Chop shallots with metal blade. Add parsley and chop. Add 2 tablespoons oil, seasonings and nuts and mix. Spread this mixture inside of trout. Reserve 1 tablespoon of stuffing for each trout for garnish. Put the 1/4 cup oil in a skillet and sauté each trout for about 8-10 minutes on each side or until nicely browned. Serve on a platter with reserved stuffing and a walnut on each trout, garnish with lemon, parsley and grapes. Can do ahead.

From: Mary lee Parrington, in "3 Rivers Cookbook III"

Poached Cod With Lemon And Capers

2 or 3 green onions, cut into 2-inch-long pieces

1 tablespoon extra-virgin olive oil

1 red onion, cut lengthwise into thin slices

2 tablespoons capers, drained well

1 carrot, cut into thin matchstick pieces

4 (4 ounce) cod fillets

2 lemons

Heat oil in a deep skillet over medium heat. Add onion and sauté 3 minutes. Add capers and sauté 1 minute. Add carrot and cook 2 min-utes. Stir in green onions. Spread vegetables evenly over bottom of skillet. Lay cod on the vegetables in skillet. Add a small amount of water just to cover the bottom of the skillet. Cover and cook until fish is just opaque in the center, about 10 minutes. Gently transfer fish to a serving platter. Top with vegetables and capers. Just before serving, squeeze the lemons over the entire dish.

From "Cooking the Whole Foods Way" by Christina Pirello.

Poached Salmon With Tomato, Caper And Scallion Sauce

skinless salmon steaks

chopped plum tomatoes (canned are fine)

capers

chopped scallions

white onion

garlic

flat leaf parsley

salt

freshly ground pepper

extra virgin olive oil

lemon juice

Combine the ingredients in a bowl. Set aside at room temperature to allow the flavors to blend. Bring 3 cups of water to boil. Place skinless salmon steaks in briskly boiling water. Bring water back to a boil (this will take about 2 minutes). Turn off the heat (or slide the pan off the heat if you have an electric range) and let the salmon steep in the hot liquid for 5 minutes. Note: The steaks will be slightly under¬done at this point. Adjust cooking time to accommodate the thickness of the steaks and personal taste preferences. Remove the steaks from the poaching liquid with a large spatula or skimmer, drain well and place each steak on a warm plate. Sponge up any liquid that collects around the steak with a paper towel and spoon the sauce over and around the steak. Serve immediately.

From: MS Dietary Home Page http:llwww.2x2.eo.nz/msl

Poached Swordfish With Lemon Parsley Sauce

In a small bowl, combine

extra virgin olive

oil

lemon juice

minced flat leaf parsley

salt and

freshly ground black pepper.

Set aside for no more than 30 minutes or the lemon juice will yel-low the parsley. Bring 3-4 cups of water to a boil in a saucepan large enough to fit the fish pieces comfortably. Holding the fish with a slotted spoon or skimmer, lower gently. into the pan and bring the water back to a boil. Reduce the heat to very low and poach the fish for 3-4 minutes until barely cooked through. Lift the fish from the water, drain thoroughly and arrange each fillet on a warm plate. Spoon the sauce over the fish and serve immedi-ately.

From: MS Dietary Home Page http:!lwww.2x2.eo.nz/msl

Cajun-Style Broiled Swordfish

1 teaspoon paprika

4 swordfish steaks, 3/4" to l" thick

1/2 teaspoon dried thyme

1/4 teaspoon garlic powder

1/4 teaspoon black pepper

1/4 teaspoon oregano

1/8 teaspoon ground red pepper

1/4 cup lemon juice

Thaw fish, if frozen. Rinse and pat dry with paper towels. For seasoning mixture, in shallow dish, stir together spices. Place lemon juice in bowl. Dip steaks in juice, then coat lightly with seasoning mixture. Preheat broiler. Spray unheated rack of pan with non-stick spray. Arrange seasoned fish on rack. Broil 4 inches from heat until fish flakes easily with fork (4 to 6 minutes per 1/2" thickness). Turn once during broiling time.

From: http://lark.cc.ukans.edul~lashlrecipes!

Broiled Lemon Swordfish

Select pieces of fish about * pound each, no more than 1 inch thick. Preheat broiler. Brush fish with olive oil and sprinkle with salt and pepper. Place fish on a wire rack in an oven-safe dish. Broil four inch¬es from heat source for 4 minutes. Turn over carefully and broil another 4 minutes. Meanwhile, combine olive oil lemon juice minced garlic capers lemon zest in a small pan. Place over low heat and cook until heated through. Place the fish on serving plates and spoon sauce on top.

From: MS Dietary Home Page http://www.2x2.co.nzlmsl

Grilled Fish With Orange Salad

2 tablespoons finely chopped red onion

pinch of crushed red pepper

2 tablespoons extra-virgin olive oil

2 teaspoons fresh lemon juice

1/2 teaspoon pepper

3 large navel oranges

8 oil-cured black olives, pitted and coarsely chopped

1/2 cup fresh mint leaves, chopped (2 Tablespoon)

4 (1/2-inch-thick) swordfish steaks, about 6 ounce each

With a sharp knife, peel oranges, making sure to remove the white pith. Holding oranges over a medium bowl, remove sections by cutting along membranes with a small knife, letting sections fall into bowl. Stir in the olives, mint, onion, crushed pepper, 1 tablespoon of the oil and the lemon juice. Refrigerate. Heat grill to HIGH and brush with about 1/2 of the oil. Brush swordfish with the other half, and sprinkle with pepper. Grill fish 2-3 minutes on each side, or just until cooked thru. Transfer fish to serving plates, top with the orange/olive/mint salad, and serve.

From "Woman's Day Magazine" 6'/2198

Fish Burgers

240 g drained canned tuna

1/2 cup finely chopped onion

1/4 cup finely chopped red capsicum

1 egg, lightly beaten

1/4 cup finely chopped celery

1 teaspoon finely chopped fresh dill

3 teaspoons lemon juice

1 tablespoon olive oil

Combine all ingredients in a bowl. Form mixture into four equal patties. Heat oil on barbecue hot plate until hot. Barbeque tuna patties 8-10 minutes, turning once. These a really good cooked on the barbeque.

I put them in the fridge for a while before I cooked them, makes a nice change from beef burgers.

From: ynnuf@clear.net.nz (Doreen Randal) in rec.food.recipes

Easy Fish And Tomato Stew

1-pound frozen fish, either cod, sole, halibut, or Boston bluefish, thawed (chopped in 1-inch cubes)

1 tablespoon extra-virgin olive oil

2 -3 garlic crushed gloves

1 large onion-sliced in 8'ths

2-3 tomatoes(sliced)

2-3 carrots diced

2-3 celery stalks diced

2-3 cups of tomato juice (add to make consistency that you prefer)

1/4 cup chopped parsley (optional)

Salt and pepper to taste

In a non-stick pain heat oil over medium heat, cook onion and garlic until softened about 5 minutes. Add celery, carrots, tomatoes, and tomato juice. Bring to a boil. Reduce heat and simmer for five minutes. Add fish and cook until fish is opaque 20-30 minutes. Add parsley and season to taste with salt and pepper. Can be served with a salad or other vegetable.

From: MS Dietary Home Page http:!lwww.2x2.co.nzlms! Adapted by Patti Vincent

Baked Fish

Crusty Fish

4-ounce fish

1 egg

1-2 Tablespoon. water

1/4-1/3 cup nut flour

Pepper

Crack egg into small bowl and beat egg. Add water to egg and beat both together. Add a little pepper to egg mixture and beat it. Place nut flour on a plate. Dip fish in egg mixture, and dip moistened fish in nut flour. Coat fish with flour on both sides. For thicker coating, repeat above procedure. If egg is left, add nut flour until your batter is thick. Make a pancake out of it and place it in the same pan with fish.

From: Elaine at www.elainecase.com/eclowcarbrecipe.html

Louisiana Fillets

2 tablespoons olive oil (substituted for butter)

2 1/2 pounds of fish fillets-sole, trout, snapper or catfish

2 tablespoons lemon juice

3/4 tsp. lemon and pepper spice

1/8 tsp. crushed red pepper

1/8 tsp. garlic powder

Preheat oven to 350°F. Heat oil with lemon juice in a shallow pan. Coat both sides of fillets with this mix. Lay fillets side by side, overlapping slightly if necessary, in a pan. Mix spices together, and sprinkle over fil¬lets. Bake for 20-25 minutes, depending on size of fillets and type of fish (catfish bakes the longest). Also, the pan may blacken, but that's fine, the liquid will keep the fish moist. Serve immediately.

From: Susan Craig in "3 Rivers Cookbook Ill"

Flounder Fillet With Dill Vegetables

2 tablespoons olive oil (substituted for butter)

1 tsp. dill weed

2 garlic cloves, minced

1 carrot, cut in thin strips

1 fresh tomato, diced

1-pound fresh flounder filet

Heat oil in skillet over low heat. Add dill and garlic. Stir to prevent browning. Add carrots and sauté for 7 minutes. Add tomato and continue to sauté for 5 minutes. Place flounder fillet in the center of a square of foil. Pour carrot-tomato mixture over the fish. Fold foil so that fish is completely enclosed. Place in baking dish and bake for 7-10 minutes in a 325°F. oven. Serve immediately

From Catherine Connell in "3 Rivers Cookbook /ff"

Baked Haddock With Tomatoes

1-pound frozen haddock fillets, thawed

2-3 Tablespoon. olive oil

1 medium onion, chopped

1 medium green pepper, chopped

1 pound can tomatoes, chopped plus juice

2 tsp. arrowroot powder

3 Tablespoon. fresh parsley, chopped (or 1 Tablespoon. dried, but fresh is better)

1/2 tsp. dried basil

1/8 tsp. black pepper

2 tsp. lemon juice (optional if tomatoes are acidic)

Sauté onion and pepper in oil about 5 min until soft. Stir in every¬thing else except fish and lemon juice and cook over medium heat 5-10 min until it thickens. Spread half the sauce in the bottom of a 9x9" baking dish. Layer the fish on top and sprinkle with lemon juice. Top with rest of sauce. Bake uncovered 375°F. 10 min until flaky (test the fish with a fork).

Adapted from Diana Hamilton <hamilton@alumni.umbc.edu>in rec.food.recipes

Baked Salmon

Salmon Fillet

2 Tomatoes (sliced)

1 large white onion (sliced)

Extra Virgin Olive Oil

Garlic

Ginger

Chopped fresh dill

Salt and freshly ground pepper

Place salmon on a piece of tin foil large enough to wrap fish for oven. Place a layer of onions over salmon and top with sliced tomatoes, driz¬zle olive oil, garlic, ginger over fish. Salt and pepper to taste. Wrap fish and bake at 400°F. for 25 minutes or until fish is opaque.

From: MS Dietary Home Page www.2x2.eo.nz/msl

Salmon Steaks With Watercress And Dill

1 bunch watercress, washed and stems removed

1 teaspoon dill weed

4 salmon steaks (about 1 3/4 pounds)

1 tablespoon lemon juice

1 tablespoon olive oil

Put the watercress in the bottom of a 2-quart baking dish and lay the salmon steaks on top. In a small bowl, mix together the lemon juice, oil, and dill, and pour over the fish. Cover and bake at 350°F. for 30 minutes or until fish flakes easily with a fork. Note: Good hot or cold. (Serves 4)

From: the Fannie Fanner cookbook, via Vickie: <Vickie@MlSO.com WWA.COM>; Adapted by Patti Vincent

Sicilian Swordfish

garlic olive oil

whole, canned tomatoes

chopped celery,

onions currants (optional)

capers

Sicilian olives (green pitted)

Wash and dry fish and dredge in nut flour. Brown fish. In a saucepan stir. Cook on medium heat for 10 minutes. Place fish in baking dish and cover with sauce. Bake at 350°F. for 20 minutes.

From: MS Dietary Home Page www.2x2.co.nzlms/

SHELLFISH

Clams, Oysters, Mussels, and Scallops

Teesryo (Goan Clams)

2 1/4 pounds clams

3 tablespoons olive oil

4 cloves garlic, chopped

1 1/2-inch piece fresh ginger, chopped

1 medium onion, chopped

2 fresh hot green chile peppers, seeded and chopped

2 teaspoons turmeric

2 tablespoons ground coriander

1 teaspoon cayenne pepper

1 cup freshly grated coconut (you can use less)

1 tablespoon lemon juice

1 tablespoon chopped fresh coriander leaves (cilantro)

Heat the oil and fry the chopped garlic, ginger, onion, and chile peppers until the onion is golden brown. Stir in the turmeric, ground coriander, and cayenne pepper. After a few minutes add the clams. Simmer, covered, for about five minutes, by which time the clam shells should have opened. Remove from heat and put in a serving bowl. Sprinkle with the freshly grated coconut, lemon juice and fresh coriander.

From: Jennifer Freeman

Mussels In Hot Pepper Sauce

2 quarts mussels

1-2 cups water

1 tablespoon olive oil

1 large garlic clove

1/2 cup chopped onion

6-ounce tomato paste

2 1/2 cups liquid from the mussels

1/2 teaspoon oregano

1/4 teaspoon (or to taste) crushed red pepper flakes, crushed

Rinse mussels in colander several times with cold water and scrub with a stiff brush to remove sand. Place mussels in pan with 1-2 cups water; steam until open. Reserve the liquid, add enough water to make 2 1/2 cups liquid and set aside. Heat oil. Sauté garlic and onion. Add remaining ingredients and simmer 30 minutes. Put mussels, in their shells, in a shallow baking dish. Cover with sauce. Bake at 425°F. for 15 minutes. Serve on the half-shell. Note: It might be necessary to strain the reserved broth.

From: Mrs. K 8. Mellon in "Three Rivers Cookbook If"

Conch And Lobster Ceviche

2 cup Conch, cleaned & diced

2 cup Lobster, diced

1/4 cup Red onion, diced

3 Scallions, sliced

1/2 small Red pepper, diced

1/2 small Yellow pepper, diced

1/2 small Green pepper, diced

1/2 small Papaya, peeled, seeded

2 Jalapeno peppers, chopped

1/2 bunch Cilantro, chopped

1/2 bunch Basil, chopped

1/2 bunch Mint, chopped

1 tablespoon Ginger, grated

1/2 Lime, juiced

1/4 cup Rice wine vinegar

1/2 cup Olive oil

Salt & pepper, to taste

1 pinch Habanera powder

In medium bowl, combine all ingredients and mix well. Season to taste. Marinate for 3 hours in refrigerator, tossing occasionally. Just before serving, adjust seasonings. Freeze stemmed glasses and fill with ceviche. Yields 6 Servings

From: Mr. Bill in rec.food.cooking

Avocado & Scallop Ceviche

1/2 cup Lime juice

3 tablespoons Olive oil

24 Green peppercorns; crushed

Salt & pepper, to taste

3/4-pound Bay scallops, chopped

1 large Avocado; peeled

2 tablespoons Chives, chopped

40 small Mushrooms

1/4 cup Olive oil

2 tablespoons Lemon juice

1 medium Garlic clove

Combine lime juice, oil, peppercorns, salt and pepper together in a glass or ceramic bowl. Stir in the scallops, cover and refrigerate for at least 4 hours while they marinate. They should become opaque in this time. Mash the avocado until almost smooth, then add it along with the chives or scallions to the marinating scallops (do not drain them) and mix well. Set aside for at least 1/2 hour, refrigerated. About half an hour before serving the scallops, remove the stems from the mushrooms and wipe them to remove any dirt. Combine the vegetable oil, lemon juice, garlic, salt and pepper in a small bowl, and brush the insides of the mushrooms liberally with the mixture. Just before serving, drain the caps and fill with the scallop mixture. Garnish with additional chives, if desired. Yield: 8 Servings

From: Mr. Bill in rec.food.cooking

Scallops Ceviche

1-pound Scallops

1 cup Lime juice

2 Garlic cloves, minced

1 Red bell pepper, julienne

2 Green sweet chilies, julienne

1/2 bunch Coriander, chopped

1 large Tomato, cored, chopped

2 Jalapeno, chopped

1/2 cup Olive oil

Slice the scallops in thirds, cutting them in a way that preserves the shape and gives a uniform size. Place the scallops in a bowl, add lime juice and marinate for 1 hour. After an hour, add the gar¬lic, red bell pepper and sweet green chili. Mix thoroughly. Add coriander, tomato, and Jalapeno chilies. Add olive oil and mix well. Serve immediately. Do NOT keep more than 2 or 3 hours. Yield: 4 Servings

From: Mr. Bill in rec.food.cooking

SHRIMP

Grilled Shellfish Ceviche

3/4-pound Shrimp; shelled

3/4-pound Sea scallops

3/4-pound Salmon fillet

1 cup Tomatoes, diced

1 cup Mango, diced

2 Grapefruit

3 Oranges

4 Limes

1/2 cup Red onion, diced

2 Jalapeno, minced

4 cup Lime juice

1 cup Cilantro, chopped

1 tablespoon Raw Honey

Salt and pepper, to taste

In a large non-reactive bowl, combine the scallops, salmon, shrimp, tomatoes, mango, onion, jalapeno and lime juice. Marinate, refrigerat¬ed, for 3 hours. Peel and segment fruits. Remove from marinade and grill fish and shellfish, just long enough to get grill marks 30-60 sec¬onds. Cut all fish in a 1/2-inch dice. Just before serving, drain off as much lime juice as possible from the fruit, add the cilantro, honey, shellfish and salmon. Gently mix being careful not to break up the fruit and fish. Yield: 6 Servings

Adapted from: Mr. Bill in rec.food.cooking

Broiled Marinated Shrimp

16 extra-large shrimp, about 1 pound, shelled and de-veined

3/4 cup extra-virgin olive oil

3 garlic cloves, chopped

1/2 teaspoon pepper

3 lemons, cut into wedges

2 tablespoons chopped fresh rosemary or 2 teaspoons dried

Place shrimp on 4 long metal skewers, threading thru tails and body. Combine oil, garlic, rosemary, and pepper in a shallow dish. Place skewered shrimp in dish, and turn to coat well. Marinate shrimp, turning several times, for 2 hours in refrigerator. Preheat broiler. Set skewers on a baking sheet set 3 inches from the heat and broil shrimp, turning once, until lightly browned, and just opaque inside, about 5 minutes. Brush with any remaining herb oil just before serving, and pass lemon wedges on the side.

From: "365 Easy Italian Recipes" by Rick Marzullo O'Connell

Luscious Lime Shrimp

20 large shrimp (about a pound) peeled & de-veined

3 tablespoons fresh lime juice

1 green onion, chopped

2 tablespoons chopped fresh cilantro

1 teaspoon minced, seeded jalapeno

1 teaspoon olive oil

1/2 teaspoon minced garlic

1 tablespoon minced red pepper

20 cucumber slices

Stir together lime juice, green onion, cilantro, jalapeno, oil, and garlic in medium bowl. Toss the shrimp with 2 tablespoons of the dressing in another medium bowl. Cover and refrigerate shrimp for 30 minutes. Preheat broiler (or grill). Broil shrimp about 3 inches from heat for 1 1/2 minutes per side or until opaque. Immediately toss hot shrimp with the remaining dressing and red pepper and cool to room temperature. Arrange shrimp on cucumber slices.

From: http://lark.cc.ukans.edu/-lashlrecipesl

En Brochette

6 strips of bacon

12 peeled and de-veined shrimp

12 raw oysters

olive oil

Cut bacon strips in half. Hold a shrimp and oyster together and wrap with a strip of bacon. Use toothpick to hold the brochette together. Heat vegetable oil to 350°F. Drop the brochette in the oil and cook approximately 3 minutes. Remove from the oil and drain excess grease.

From: http://lark.cc.ukans.edu/-lashlrecipesl Adapted by Patti Vincent

Island Barbequed Shrimp

1-pound shrimp, jumbo or large, cleaned, tails on

2 tablespoons olive oil

1 tablespoon garlic, finely minced

1 tablespoon rosemary, chopped fresh

1/2 teaspoon thyme, chopped fresh

1/4 teaspoon cayenne pepper, or to taste

1/4 teaspoon salt

2 limes, halved

Combine all except shrimp and limes. Marinate at room temperature for 1 hour. Heat a dry skillet over medium-high heat. When skillet is hot, lay shrimp in pan. Cook shrimp 2-4 minutes per side. Brush with remaining marinade before turning. Serve with lime.

From:johnstoc@addor.medium.unc.edu (Charlie Johnston) 29 Jun 1994. Posted to rec.food.recipes by Doreen Randal

Curried Shrimp

Verra Moolee (Kerala Prawns In Coconut Milk)

2 1/4 pounds large prawns (shrimp), shelled and de-veined

3 1/2-ounce olive or coconut oil

1 medium onion, finely chopped

4 cloves garlic, minced

1 1/2-inch piece fresh ginger, minced

4 fresh hot green chile peppers, seeded and minced

2 tablespoons ground coriander

1 teaspoon turmeric

16-ounce coconut milk

2/3 cup fresh coriander leaves, chopped

Heat the oil and fry the onion until golden brown. Add the garlic, gin¬ger, and chile peppers and cook with the onions for about 5 minutes. Stir in the spices and after a few seconds pour in the coconut milk. Simmer for approximately 15 minutes until the coconut milk has thickened and slightly reduced. Add the prawns and cook them gently in the spiced coconut sauce until done, about 5 minutes. Just before serving stir in the chopped coriander leaves.

From: Jennifer Freeman

Shrimp Curry

2 tablespoons olive oil

1 medium onion, finely chopped

1 (8 ounce) can tomato sauce

2 teaspoons minced fresh ginger (essential)

2 cloves garlic, minced

1/2 teaspoon cumin 1/2 teaspoon coriander

1/2 teaspoon turmeric lime juice

1 package (6 ounce) frozen shelled, de-veined shrimp, thawed,

OR an equivalent amount of fresh or canned shrimp

Heat oil and sauté onion at low temperature until golden brown. Add tomato sauce, ginger, garlic, and spices. Bring to simmer. Add a little water if too thick. Add shrimp to sauce. Simmer 5 minutes. Add a little lime juice just before serving.

From: Barbara Schrading in "The Great Tomato Patch Cookbook"

Quick Shrimp Curry

1 onion wedged

1-2 cups frozen shrimp

cayenne pepper

garlic

curry powder

2 cups frozen vegetables, I used broccoli and yellow (summer) squash

walnut oil

1/4-1/2 cup pure coconut milk

Stir fry ingredients in walnut oil and a little water until thawed through and almost hot add coconut milk and more curry powder, stir to coat and cook until heated through. Serve. Takes about 15 minutes, max. A quick recipe for when you want something "dif-ferent" but don't have all day and nothing is thawed. Obviously this also works with all kinds of Diet Evolution correct vegetables and meats.

From: Kathleen <Yoeschucho@AOL.COM>

LOBSTER

Coconut Lobster

Meat of 4 medium-sized cooked lobsters, shelled and cut into chunks

1/2 cup nutmilk (optional)

1 cup coconut milk

1 small onion, finely chopped

2 scallions, finely chopped

2 springs thyme

2 tablespoons curry powder

Salt and freshly ground white or black pepper to taste

Dash cayenne pepper

Fresh lime or lemon wedges

Preheat oven to 400°F. Mix the nutmilk and coconut milk together. Heat in a large saucepan over moderate heat. Add the onion, scallions, thyme, and curry powder. Stir and cook for about 5 min. Add the lob¬ster chunks, salt, pepper and cayenne. Cook slowly for 7-8 min. so that all flavors are well blended. Remove to a baking dish. Bake for about 15 min. or until lobster is browned. Serve with lime or lemon wedges. Serve in the lobster shells! Serves 4

Adapted from: E.A.M.L.v. Loen in rec.food.recipes

Broiled Lobster Tails

4 frozen lobster tails

2 quarts boiling water

1 tablespoon salt

1/4 cup lemon juice

Drop frozen lobster tails in boiling water; add salt and lemon juice; heat to boiling again. Reduce heat, cover and simmer 20 minutes. Drain. With a sharp knife or kitchen scissors, remove soft shell-like covering on underside of tail. Drizzle olive oil over lobster meat; sprin¬kle with paprika. Place lobster on rack 4-6 inches from broiler. Broil 6 minutes. Serve in shell.

Modified from one in rec.food.recipes by: food.chal@simpleinlemel.com

EGGS

Baked Eggs In Bacon Rings

6 strips nitrite-free bacon or fresh pork side melted bacon fat for brushing tins

4 slices tomato, each about 1/2 inch thick

4 eggs

pepper to taste

chopped onions (optional)

Preheat the oven to 325°F. Cook bacon in a skillet over medium heat until it begins to shrivel, about 3 minutes. Remove from heat. Brush 4 cups in a muffin tin or 4 small ramekins with bacon fat. Place a tomato slice in the bottom of each cup. Circle the inside of each cup with 1 1/2 strips of bacon. Break an egg into each muf¬fin cup and season with pepper. Can add chopped onions. Fill any unused tins with water to protect them from burning. Bake in the oven for 20 minutes. To serve, loosen the edges of the eggs with spatula and transfer the eggs to plates. Serves 2.

Adapted from Dr. Atkins' Quick and Easy New Diet Cookbook

Puffy Omelet

4 eggs, separated

1/4 cup water

1/8 teaspoon pepper

1 tablespoons butter

Beat egg whites and water in small mixer bowl until stiff but not dry. Beat egg yolks and pepper in another bowl until very thick and lemon colored, about 5 minutes. Fold into egg whites. Heat butter in 10-inch ovenproof skillet until hot enough to sizzle drop of water. Pour omelet mixture into skillet; level surface gently. Reduce heat. Cook slowly until puffy and light brown on the bottom, about 5 minutes. (Lift omelet at edge to look at color.) Cook uncovered in 325°F. oven until knife inserted in center comes out clean, 12 to 15 minutes. Tilt skillet; slip pancake turner or spatula under omelet to loosen. Fold omelet in half, being careful not to break it. Slip onto warm plate.

From Pam at http://www.ilovejesus.comllotllocarb/

Cherokee Green Onions And Eggs

3 tablespoons bacon fat

2 bunches of wild green onions, whites and crisp green tops, trimmed and sliced in 1/4" rounds, or you may substitute shallots, chives, garlic (or "Chinese") chives, young leeks, or any combination for as much as half of the green onions.

1/4 cup water

7 large eggs or 6 jumbo eggs

pepper (optional)

Heat bacon fat in a large heavy skillet over medium heat. Add green onions and turn in fat to coat. Lower heat, cover, and simmer for about 5 minutes. Uncover and add water. Cook over low heat for about 10 minutes more, stirring occasionally, until green onions are tender but not brown. If water is all absorbed, add more by tablespoons. Break eggs into the skillet and stir with a fork until they are scrambled. Raise heat to medium. Continue to stir until eggs are as cooked as desired. When they are nearly done, adjust the seasonings. Serves 3-4.

Adapted /ram "Regional American Classics"; California Culinary Academy.

Myra's Chopped Egg And Onion

12 hard-boiled eggs, peeled

1 small onion, diced fine

1/3 cup schmaltz

White pepper to taste

Chop the eggs to your own preference (I prefer pretty finely chopped eggs). Set aside. Sauté the onion in the schmaltz until it starts to brown. Add the onion and schmaltz to the chopped eggs and mix well. Add pepper to taste, and chill. Makes about 4-6 servings. Note: You can spread this on celery! You can substitute vegetable oil for the schmaltz.

From Betty <lguyer@JUNO.COM>

Myra's Chopped Mushrooms, Eggs And Onion

1 medium onion, finely diced

1/4 cup schmaltz or vegetable oil

10-12 medium white mushrooms, finely chopped

12 hard-boiled eggs, peeled and finely chopped

Freshly ground black pepper to taste

Sauté the onion in the schmaltz or oil until golden brown. Add the mushrooms and sauté another 5 minutes or so, stirring frequently, until mushrooms are softened and turned dark. Remove from heat and let cool. Mix together with the eggs and pepper. Chill until ready to serve. Makes 6 to 8 servings. Note: I really like this as an appetizer.

From Betty <fguyer@JUNO.COM>

My Favorite Dinner Omelet

1 cup of chopped fresh spinach

4 chopped green onions

1 clove of fresh chopped garlic

1/2 cup of Portobello mushrooms

3 eggs

1/4 cup V-8 juice

pepper, cayenne pepper to taste

Sauté chopped vegetables in hot olive oil. Beat eggs, V-8 juice and seasonings in bowl. Pour eggs over sauteed vegetables and cook until firm. Flip omelet and cook other side until firm. Garnish with fresh tomato slices and serve.

From Binnie <.betten+@pitt.edu>

Quiche Crust, Or Nutty Nut Patty

1 cup sunflower seeds

1 cup almonds

3 carrots

1 garlic clove

1 beet

2 celery stalks

1/2 onion

1/2 cup parsley

lemon juice

Soak sunflower seeds and almonds separately for eight to 12 hours and rinse. Alternate putting the sunflower seeds, almonds, carrots, garlic and beets through the food processor or blender and into a bowl. Stir the mixture adding finely diced celery, onion, bell peppers and parsley, spicing with lemon juice to taste. Form into a crust shape or patties 1/2-inch-thick by two to three inches round. Warm in dehydrator at 105°F. until warm or a low temperature oven at 200°F.

From Susan <Scarmack@WIC.ORG>

VEGETABLES

Country-Style Greens

1 tablespoon lard or rendered bacon fat

1 medium onion, minced

2 cups water pepper

2 bunches (or about 2 pounds) of fresh collard, turnip, or mustard greens

1/4-pound good quality bacon or ham, cut in 1/2-inch pieces, or 1/2-pound ordinary sliced bacon or ham

Trim away and discard the tough stems of the greens. To loosen grit, place the leaves and the remaining tender stems (you should have about 2 quarts) in a large bowl, cover with lukewarm water, and soak for 5 minutes. Rinse several times in lukewarm water to wash away any remaining sand. Melt lard in a large heavy nonreactive pot with a lid. Do not use an aluminum pot, if possible, use one with an enamel coating. Add onions and bacon. Fry together over medium-high heat, stirring often, until onions wilt and bacon starts to brown, about 5 minutes. Add greens and the water and bring to a boil over high heat. Cover, lower heat to medium, and cook until greens are tender, with just a little crunch, about 20 minutes. Uncover, raise heat to high, and boil off some of the excess water, about 5 minutes. Add pepper to taste, and serve hot, it should be slightly soupy. Serves 6.

Adapted from "Regional American Classics". California Culinary Academy.

Lettuce And Bacon

6 small heads of romaine lettuce

1/2-pound bacon, diced

1 large onion, minced

1 large tomato, peeled and seeded (optional)

fresh ground pepper

sprinkling of a favorite herb: basil, thyme or marjoram

chicken broth or water (if necessary to prevent scorching)

Trim the romaine heads, but leave them whole. Wash thru several changes of cold water, shake dry, Plunge the lettuce into a large saucepan filled with boiling water, and cook for about 2 minutes. Do not overcook, the lettuce must remain firm. Drain and lay in a strainer to allow the lettuce to drip excess moisture. Dry between paper towels. In a fry pan, cook bacon until crisp. Pour off about 2/3 of the fat in the pan. Add the onion and the tomato, and cook, stirring constantly, until onion is tender. Add the lettuce, season with pepper, and sprinkle with your herbs. Cook covered over low heat for about 10 minutes, check for dryness, if necessary, add a little broth or water, 1-2 tablespoons at a time, to prevent scorching. The cooked lettuce should be dry. Serve very hot, 4-6 servings.

From "Nika Hazelton's Way with Vegetables"

Roman Spinach

3 pounds spinach, washed and trimmed

2-3 tablespoons olive oil

1/2 cup pignolias (pine nuts)

1 garlic clove, mashed

2 teaspoons lemon juice or to taste

pepper

Cut any large spinach leaves into pieces. Heat the oil in a deep-frying pan. Cook the nuts, stirring constantly until they are golden. Add the spinach, garlic, lemon juice, and pepper to taste. Cook covered, shaking the pan to prevent sticking, for about 4 minutes, or until barely tender. Serve very hot, 4 servings.

Broccoli With Golden Garlic And Lemon

1 bunch broccoli, about 1 pound

1/4 cup extra virgin olive oil

3 garlic cloves, cut into thin slivers

1/8 teaspoon pepper

3 tablespoons fresh lemon juice

Cook broccoli in a large saucepan of boiling water 5-6 minutes, or until crisp tender. Drain in a colander. Arrange on a serving dish and cover to keep warm. In a small frying pan, warm olive oil over low heat. Stir in garlic and cook slowly until golden brown, be careful not to burn the garlic, about 1-2 minutes. Add pepper and lemon juice. Pour over broccoli.

From "365 Easy Italian Recipes" by Rick Marzullo O'Connell

Broccoli With Artichoke Hearts

1 head broccoli, cut into flowerets

1/2 teaspoon extra virgin olive oil

pinch of minced dried hot chile or to taste

2-3 cloves garlic, minced

1 (6 ounce) jar marinated artichoke hearts, drained and halved

juice of 1 lime, or 1 lemon

Bring a small amount of water to a boil and steam broccoli flowerets until bright green and crisp-tender, about 5 minutes. Plunge into cold water to stop the cooking process, drain and set aside. Heat oil in a skillet over medium heat. Add hot chile and garlic. Cook 1 minute. Stir in artichoke hearts and cook abut 3 minutes. Remove from heat and stir in broccoli and lime or lemon juice. Transfer to a serving bowl, and serve immediately.

From "Cooking the Whole Foods Way" by Christina Pirel/o.

Olive Broccoli

1 head broccoli

1 teaspoon extra virgin olive oil

juice and grated zest of 1 lemon

1/2 cup oil-cured olives, pitted and minced

1 red bell pepper, roasted over an open flame, peeled, seeded and diced

Split broccoli lengthwise into spears, trimming off any coarse stems and leaves. Bring a small amount of water to a boil over high heat. Add broccoli and steam until bright green and crisp-tender, about 4 min¬utes. Drain and transfer to a bowl. Immediately drizzle lightly with oil and toss gently. Stir in lemon juice and zest, bell pepper, and minced olives and turn the ingredients gently to combine. Arrange on a plat¬ter and serve warm.

From "Cooking the Whole Foods Way" by Christina Pirello.

Red Cabbage With Chestnuts

1-pound fresh chestnuts

2 tablespoons olive oil

1 large onion, thinly sliced

1 2-pound head red cabbage, cored, thinly sliced

1/2 cup red wine vinegar (or a DE substitute?)

6 tablespoons water

3 tablespoons honey

In typical Alsatian fashion, this cabbage has a delicious sweet-and-¬sour flavor. Preheat oven to 400°F. Using small knife, cut an X in each chestnut. Place in roasting pan. Bake until shells loosen, about 35 minutes. Cool slightly. Remove hard shell and brown skin from each nut. Set aside. Heat oil in large pot over medium low heat. Add onion; sauté until soft, about 5 minutes. Add cabbage, vinegar, water and sugar. Cover; cook until cabbage is tender, stirring occasionally, about 40 minutes. Add nuts; cook until warm, about 10 minutes longer. Season with pepper.

From Bon Appetit December 1997

Grilled Harvest Vegetables

1 small cabbage, cored

2 tablespoons olive oil

1/2 to 1 teaspoon onion powder, optional

1/8 to 1/4 teaspoon pepper

4 medium carrots, cut into 1-inch pieces

2 celery ribs, cut into 1-inch pieces

1 small onion, cut into wedges

1/2-pound whole fresh mushrooms

1 small green pepper, cut into pieces

4 bacon strips, cooked and crumbled, optional

Cut cabbage into 6 wedges; spread oil on cut sides. Place cabbage on a piece of heavy-duty foil, about 24" by 18". Sprinkle with onion powder, if desired, and pepper. Arrange remaining vegetables and bacon (if desired) around cabbage. Seal the foil tightly. Grill, covered, over medium-high heat for 30 minutes or until vegetables are tender, turning occasionally.

From: Quick Cooking, Sept/Oct 1998: Adapted by Patti Vincent

Indian Cauliflower And Scallions With Black Mustard Seeds

1 head cauliflower, about 1 1/4 pounds

2 small bunches of scallions

2 teaspoons black mustard seeds (found in Indian or Middle Eastern markets or spice shops)

2 teaspoons cumin seeds

1 teaspoon fennel seeds

1/2 teaspoon turmeric

1/3 cup warm water (105°F.)

1/4 cup olive oil

1/3 cup chopped fresh coriander or 8 fresh curry leaves

Separate and cut the cauliflower into 1-inch florets. Peel the cauliflower stem and cut into thin slices. Set aside. Trim the scallions and chop them, including the entire green part. Set aside. Measure out the spices and place them, as well as the water, right next to the stove. Heat the oil in a wok or a sauté pan over high heat. When the oil is hot, add the mustard, cumin, and fennel. Keep a pot lid handy since the seeds may splatter and sputter when added. When the seeds stop sputtering, add the turmeric and immediately add the cauliflower. Stir-fry the cauliflower until it's evenly coated with spice-infused oil. Add the scallions and water; mix and cover with a lid. Cook over medium heat and toss a couple times until the cauliflower is soft, about 10 minutes. Uncover, fold in the coriander, and continue stir-frying until excess moisture evaporates and the cauliflower looks glazed, about 5 min¬utes. Turn off the heat and serve. Serves 4

From: "The Frugal Gourmet On Our Immigrant Ancestors" by Jeff Smith

Ratatouille

1 small eggplant

1/4 cup olive oil pepper

4 tomatoes, chopped

2 small zucchinis

1 medium onion, sliced

1/4 cup parsley, minced

2 cloves garlic, minced

1 green pepper, sliced

Peel eggplant, slice 1/4" thick. Cover and weigh down. Let stand for 30 minutes while you prepare other veggies. The drain the eggplant, dry on towel, cut slices into quarters. Heat half the oil, fry the egg-plant and remove. Add remaining oil, fry garlic, onions and peppers until softened. Place tomatoes on top of onions, cover pan, and cook 5 minutes. Take cover off, raise heat, cook 5 minutes more without cover. Stir in minced parsley. Arrange a layer of tomato mixture on the bottom of a 2-quart casserole dish. Cover with a layer of sliced zucchini, and half the eggplant. Put half of the rest of the tomatoes on, then the remaining eggplant and the rest of the zucchini. Finish with layer of tomatoes. Bake about 30 minutes at 350°F.

From "The New Fann Vegetarian Cookbook"

Baked Whole Garlic

4 whole heads of garlic

1/2 cup olive oil (approximately.)

pepper

1 teaspoon thyme leaves

Preheat the oven to 275°F. Slice the top (1/4 inch) from the heads of garlic and rub to remove some of the papery skin from the outside, taking care not to separate the cloves. Put the heads in a baking dish that will just hold them. Pour the olive oil over each, add the pepper and thyme. Cover and bake for about 30 minutes. Remove the cover and continue to bake for about 1-1 1/2 hours longer. The garlic mellows and turns creamy as it bakes, and should be very tender. To eat, squeeze one clove at a time out of the skins.

From the "Fannie Fanner cookbook," via Vickie <vickie@MJSO.com WWA.COM>

Mushrooms A La Provençale

1/4 cup olive oil

1-pound mushrooms, thickly sliced or quartered

2 whole garlic cloves

pepper

1/2 teaspoon dried thyme, or 3 sprigs fresh thyme

1/2 cup minced parsley

juice of 1/2 lemon

Heat oil in a heavy pan with a close-fitting lid. Add the mushrooms, garlic, and pepper, and thyme. Cook covered over medium to high heat for 5-7 minutes, shaking the pan very frequently to prevent sticking. Then sprinkle with parsley and lemon juice, and serve very hot.

From "Nika Hazelton's Way with Vegetables"

Mushroom Pate

1 teaspoon extra virgin olive oil

4-5 shallots, minced

2-3 garlic clove, minced

juice of 1 lemon

fresh parsley for garnish

1-pound button mushrooms, brushed clean and diced

2 tablespoons pecans, lightly dry-roasted in a skillet over medium heat about 3 minutes and minced

Heat oil in a skillet over medium heat. Add shallots, garlic and cook until fragrant, about 3 minutes. Add mushrooms and cook, stirring, 10-15 minutes, until mushroom liquid has been reabsorbed into the vegetables. Transfer the cooked mushroom mixture to a food processor and puree until smooth. Spoon into a bowl and gently fold in pecans and lemon juice. Transfer to a small serving bowl, cover and refrigerate to cool completely before serving, garnished with fresh parsley.

From "Cooking the 147wle Foods Way" by Christina Pirello.

Marinated Mushrooms

2 pounds of fresh mushrooms

1/2 cup lemon juice

1 cup olive oil

3 medium onions, thinly sliced

1/4 teaspoon pepper

1 teaspoon dry mustard

1 teaspoon thyme

1/2 teaspoon oregano

1 teaspoon basil

2 teaspoons honey (substitute for sugar

Combine all ingredients and cook for 5-10 minutes over medium heat. Cool. Cover and refrigerate overnight.

From Laurie M. Lijoi in "3 Rivers Cookbook III"

Whole Roasted Onions

Prep Time: about 1-1/2 hours, roast with your turkey. Place 5 or 6 unpeeled onions (1/2 pound each) in a 9"x13" pan. Bake in a 325°F. oven until onions give readily when gently squeezed, about 1-1/2 hours. Lift from pan and cut each onion in half lengthwise. Season to taste.

From: Sunset, Nov. 1998

Braised Onions, Shallots And Leeks

1 teaspoon extra virgin olive oil

3 red onions, cut into thick wedges

fresh basil, minced, or dried basil

juice of 1 lime

4 or 5 shallots, halved

3 Vidalia (or yellow) onions, cut into thick wedges

3 leeks, cut lengthwise, rinsed well and sliced into 2" lengths

Heat oil in deep skillet over low heat. Add onions and cook, stirring until they begin to soften, about 10 minutes. Add shallots and cook, stirring, 4-5 minutes. Add leeks and cook, stirring, until bright green and tender, 5 minutes. Add a little water and a sprinkling of basil. Cover and simmer until any remaining liquid has been absorbed. Remove from heat and stir in lime juice.

From "Cooking the Whole Foods Way" by Christina Pirello.

Italian Onion Antipasto

4 large onions, peeled and ends removed

4 cloves garlic, peeled

4 pinches of dried thyme

extra virgin olive oil

4-6 leaves of romaine or red leaf lettuce

Preheat oven to 375°F. (190°C). Lightly oil a shallow casserole dish. Stand the onions on their root ends in the casserole dish. Press a clove of garlic and a pinch of thyme into the center of each onion. Drizzle with a little olive oil. Add just enough water to cover the bottom of the baking dish, cover, and bake 40 minutes. Remove cover and return casserole dish to oven for about 10 minutes or until onions are tender. Remove onions from casserole, slice into thick wedges, and serve 2 or 3 hot wedges on lettuce.

From "Cooking the Whole Foods Way" by Christina Pirello.

Roasted Yellow Peppers

4 large yellow bell peppers, about 2 pounds

3 tablespoons extra virgin olive oil

2 tablespoons shredded fresh basil, or 1 1/2 tablespoons chopped fresh parsley and 1 tsp dried basil

pepper to taste

Preheat oven to 475°F. Set peppers on a baking sheet, and brush with 1 tablespoon oil to coat lightly. Bake, turning once or twice, for 20 minutes, or until skins begin to blister. Place peppers in a brown bag or plastic bag to steam for 10 minutes. Pull skins from peppers. Remove stems, seeds, and membranes. Tear peppers into 4 to 6 pieces each. Lay roasted peppers flat on a serving plate. In a small bowl, mix the remaining 2 tablespoons olive oil, basil and slat/pepper. Pour over roasted peppers.

From "365 Easy Italian Recipes" by Rick Marzullo O'Connell

Pepperoni Al Forno

4 very large green, red or yellow sweet peppers, peeled and seeded

2 large ripe tomatoes, peeled

1/2 cup black olives, pitted and coarsely chopped

1 large onion, thinly sliced

2 garlic cloves, chopped

4 anchovies, drained and chopped (optional)

pepper

1 cup parsley sprigs

1/2 cup fresh minced basil or 2 tablespoons dried basil

1/4 to 1/2 cup olive oil

Cut peppers into wedge strips. Cut tomatoes into wedges the size of the pepper strip. Put peppers, tomatoes, olives, onion, garlic, and anchovies into a baking dish. Season with pepper. Mince together the parsley and basil, and sprinkle over the vegetables. Then sprinkle with olive oil. Cook at 350°F. for about 30 minutes.

From "Nika Hazelton's Way with Vegetables"

Provencal Vegetables

3 tablespoons virgin olive oil

1 medium red bell pepper, finely diced

1 medium zucchini, finely diced

1 medium yellow squash, finely diced

In a large skillet, heat the oil over medium-high heat until shimmering. Add the pepper, zucchini, and squash and sauté until tender, 3 to 4 minutes.

To serve:

1 cup greens of your choice [I used mesclun]

About 1/2 cup Lime Dressing [see recipe in Salad Dressings]

When read to serve, toss the greens with 1/4 cup of the Lime Dressing and the Provencal vegetables. Divide among 4 plates, arrange 1 quail breast and 2 legs around the greens, and drizzle with additional Lime Dressing.

From: "French Food American Accent" by Debra Ponzek via Kay in RFC

Sweet 'N Crunchy Zucchini Chips

1. Slice Zucchini into 1/4 inch "chips"

2. Dry the chips in a food dehydrator. (105°F. recommended)

3. Eat the chips plain, dip into avocado or guacamole, or add to cold raw soups or salads.

From David Klein, http://www.living-foods.com/livingnutrition

MEAT SOUPS

Homemade Beef Broth

4 pounds meaty beef soup bones (beef shanks or short ribs)

3 medium carrots, cut into chunks

3 celery ribs, cut into chunks

2 medium onions, quartered

1/2 cup warm water

3 bay leaves

3 garlic cloves

8-10 whole peppercorns

3-4 sprigs fresh parsley

1 teaspoon EACH dried thyme, marjoram, and oregano

3 quarts cold water

Place soup bones in a large roasting pan. Bake, uncovered, at 450°F. for 30 minutes. Add carrots, celery and onions. Bake 30 minutes longer; drain fat. With a slotted spoon, transfer bones and vegetables to a soup kettle. Add warm water to the roasting pan; stir to loosen browned bits from pan. Transfer pan juices to the kettle. Add seasonings and enough cold water just to cover. Slowly bring to a boil, about 30 minutes. Reduce heat; simmer, uncovered, for 4-5 hours, skimming the surface as foam rises. If necessary, add hot water during the first 2 hours to keep ingredients covered. Set beef bones aside until cool enough to handle. Remove meat form bones; give bones to favorite dog, save meat for your own use. Strain broth, discarding vegetables and seasonings. Refrigerate for 8 hours or overnight. Skim fat from surface. Makes about 2-1/2 quarts

From: Quick Cooking, Sept/Oct 1998

CHICKEN SOUPS

Cock-A-Leekie (Rooster Soup)

1 3-pound chicken, cut up

2 carrots, coarsely chopped

1 onion, quartered

1/2 teaspoon fresh ground pepper

6-8 prunes (optional)

1 bouquet garni (4 parsley sprigs, 1/4 teaspoon dried thyme, 1 bay leaf, and 8 peppercorns tied in cheesecloth)

5-6 medium leeks, the white part only, well-rinsed, and cut into 1/2" pieces

1 tablespoon chopped fresh parsley

Place chicken in a large Dutch oven or stockpot. Pour in 2 quarts of water, and bring to a boil over high heat; skim off foam as it collects. Add carrots, onion, bouquet garni, and pepper. Reduce heat, and simmer 45 minutes, until chicken is falling off the bones. Remove chicken and let cool; remove skin and bones; cut meat into bite-sized pieces. Strain stock into a large bowl, discard vegetables and bouquet garni. Skim off fat. In a large saucepan, heat a couple tablespoons of olive oil. Add leeks, cover and cook 10 minutes, until soft. Pour reserved stock over leeks. Bring to a boil, reduce heat, and cook 15 minutes. Add chicken and prunes, simmer 15 minutes. Season with pepper to taste. Add parsley and serve.

From "365 Ways to Cook Chicken" by Cheryl Sedaker.

Homemade Chicken Broth

2-1/2 pounds bony chicken pieces

2 celery ribs with leaves, cut into chunks

2 medium carrots, cut into chunks

2 medium onions, quartered

2 bay leaves

1/2 teaspoon dried rosemary, crushed

1/2 teaspoon dried thyme

8-10 whole peppercorns

2 quarts cold water

Place all ingredients in a soup kettle or Dutch oven. Slowly bring to a boil; reduce heat. Skim foam. Cover and simmer for 2 hours. Set chicken aside until cool enough to handle. Remove meat from bones. Discard bones; save meat for another use. Strain broth, discarding vegetables and seasonings. Refrigerate for 8 hours or overnight. Skim fat from surface. Makes about 6 cups of chicken broth.

From: Quick Cooking, Sept/Oct 1998

Tom Kha Kai (Thai Coconut Chicken Soup)

4 cubed skinless boneless chicken breast halves

2 cups coconut milk (canned, in the Oriental foods section)

1 teaspoon Laos powder (from an Oriental grocery)

2 chopped green onions

4 chopped serrano chiles

2 teaspoons powdered lemon grass (from an Oriental grocery; or use fresh lemon grass)

1 juiced lime

Bring 1 cup coconut milk to boil. Add chicken, lemon grass, and Laos. Cover and simmer until chicken is tender.** Add remaining 1 cup coconut milk, green onions and chilis. DO NOT BOIL. Stir in lime juice just before serving. **Or, cook chicken with coconut milk and seasonings in the microwave at about 50% power for 20 minutes. Makes the broth especially rich!

From: gilcat2@aol.com (Gilcat2) in rec.food.recipes; Adapted by Patti Vincent

FISH SOUPS

Thai Hot & Sour Shrimp Soup

1 tablespoon olive oil

Shells from shrimp (see below)

8 cups chicken stock

3 stalks lemon grass, cut into 1" lengths

4 kaffir lime leaves (can be found in Thai and Chinese markets, often frozen)

1 teaspoon lime zest

2 green Serrano chiles, slivered

2 pounds fresh shrimp, approximately 20 count per pound, shelled and deveined

1 tablespoon coconut milk

1/2 teaspoon salt

juice of 2 limes

1 red Serrano chili, slivered

2 tablespoons coriander leaves (cilantro), coarsely chopped

3 green onions (including some green), coarsely chopped

Heat the oil in a saucepan and fry the shells until they turn pink. Add the chicken stock, lemon grass, lime leaves, lime rind, and green chilis. Bring to a boil, cover, reduce heat and simmer for 20 minutes. Strain the mixture through a sieve, return the liquid to a saucepan and bring to a boil.

Add the shrimp to this boiling "stock" and cook them for 2- 3 minutes. Reduce heat to simmer and add the coconut milk, salt and lime juice. Stir and immediately remove from heat to prevent overcooking. Pour the soup in a tureen or ladle into bowls, sprinkle with red chilis, coriander leaves and green onions. Serve piping-hot.

From: "The Original Thai Cookbook" by Jennifer Brennan; Adapted by Patti Vincent

Hans' Fish Soup

I made salmon soup the other day. I boiled the bones and fins and tail (I had bought the tail half of a salmon) for I guess an hour. Then I strained to get the broth separated from bones and other, cut some of the salmon filets in small pieces, added to the broth together with some fresh onion and other green spicy things and boiled for a few minutes. Tasted very good. I guess you can boil fish heads for a few minutes to be able to peel away the good meat pieces, to put aside when boiling the boney and fatty parts for quite a while, then putting the meat back into the soup just to warm before serving (to not overcook the meat).

From Hans <hans-k@ALGONET.SE>

VEGETABLE SOUPS

Vegetable Cabbage Soup

soup bone

1/2-pound stewing beef

3 quarts water

1-2 bay leaves

1 small head of cabbage

4 medium to large carrots

4-6 stalks of celery

1 medium-large onion

1 can tomatoes, cut up

6-ounce tomato juice

Put a soup bone and 1/2-pound stewing beef in a large pot and fill with 3 quarts water. Add bay leaves. Simmer 2-3 hours, Skim top from time to time. Chop coarsely the cabbage, carrots, celery and onion. Remove bone from soup and add vegetables. Cook 30 minutes. Add tomatoes and tomato juice. Bring to a boil again and serve.

From: Mrs. David S. Schaff III, in "Seasoned in Sewickley"

Cream Of Cauliflower Soup

a large head of cauliflower

2-3 stalks celery

1 carrot

2 cloves garlic

1-2 onions

1-2 teaspoons ground cumin

1/2 teaspoon pepper

a few sprigs of parsley

1/4 teaspoon sage (or your favorite blend of herbs; spices)

Chop head of cauliflower (save a handful of tiny flowerets for a raw garnish) and put in a soup pot. Chop; add stalks celery, carrot, gar¬lic and onions. Add spices. Barely cover with water, bring to boil and simmer until veggies are tender. Blend the contents of the pot and adjust seasonings to taste. Add a little hot water if the soup is too thick. Serve garnished with raw flowerets. Serving suggestion: Serve with a steak, plus a spinach/lettuce and mushroom salad garnished with grated carrot and parsley. You can use the same basic recipe for Cream of Broccoli or Cream of Asparagus Soup. You won't miss the fact that is no actual cream in the soup, given the thick consistency and rich flavor of the main veggie. You can also add chopped, cooked meat for a quick lunch.

From: Chris <fincham@PETERBORO.NET>

Cream Of Mushroom Soup

1 avocado

1 tomato

1 cup hot water

1 red sweet pepper (diced)

1 cup mushrooms (sliced)

1 little onion (diced)

1 clove of garlic

Juice of 1/2 grapefruit,

chopped basil

Blend avocado, grapefruit juice, garlic and hot water. This time the consistency of your soup should be thicker and creamier. Then add sliced mushrooms, sweet pepper, onion and basil. You may choose any of your favorite vegetables as an addition to your soup.

By Tatiana Kozlova at www.rawtimes.com

Gazpacho

4 ripe tomatoes, quartered

1 small onion, coarsely chopped

1 clove garlic, peeled

1 cup tomato juice

2 tablespoons lemon juice

pepper to taste

cayenne, if you want to

1 sprig fresh parsley

4 ice cubes

1 medium cucumber, peeled and coarsely chopped

Blend all ingredients in blender or food processor, until vegetables are small but NOT pureed.

From: "Cooking Healthy with One Foot out the Door"

Scallion Chive Soup

1/2 cup zucchini, shredded

1/2 cup shallots, chopped

1 clove garlic, minced

3 teaspoons olive oil

1 cup scallions, chopped

1/2 cup chives, chopped

2 cup chicken broth

1/2 cup water

In saucepan, cook zucchini, shallots, and garlic in oil over moder¬ately low heat. Stir occasionally until shallots are tender (about 5 minutes.). Add scallions and all but 2 tablespoons chives. Cook, stirring, until scallions are softened, about 2 minutes. Stir in broth and water. Simmer 2 minutes. In a blender, puree mixture. Pour soup through a fine sieve into clean pan, pressing hard on solids and discarding them. Heat soup over moderate heat, stirring until hot. Season to taste. Stir in remaining chives.

From: hllp://lark.cc.ukans.edu/-lash/recipesl; Adapted by P. Vincent

Zucchini Soup

1 large onion, chopped

2 tablespoons olive oil

2 cups chicken broth

8 cups diced zucchini

1/8 teaspoon garlic powder

1/8 teaspoon celery

salt

dash of pepper

1/4 cup parsley leaves

In a pan, sauté onion in oil until tender. Add remaining ingredients except parsley. Cook over medium heat about 5 minutes or until zucchini is tender. Carefully pour into blender or food processor, and add parsley and whirl at high speed until smooth. May be thinned with additional chicken broth. Serve hot or cold. Can be frozen.

From: Mrs. Wythe B. Weathers, in "Seasoned in Sewickley"

SALADS

Fresh Spinach Salad

1-pound fresh spinach, washed, drained and torn into desired pieces

1 can sliced water chestnuts

1-pound fresh mushrooms, sliced thinly

1/2-pound bacon, cooked and crumbled

4 hardboiled eggs, sliced

Make sure spinach has been well drained and isn't watery. Combine all above salad ingredients in a large bowl. (I usually toss the spinach, mushrooms, and water chestnuts together then top with bacon and sliced hardboiled eggs as garnish until time to serve.) Chill. This is also another "most requested" dish at family dinners and is a wonderful change from a plain iceberg lettuce salad. Leftovers don't keep well; spinach tends to wilt down. So, eat it all at the first serving or shortly thereafter.

From: cyndeed@aol.com (Cyndee D) in rec.food.recipes

Grapefruit Walnut Salad

2 tablespoons agar-agar flakes or gelatin

1 1/2 cup boiling water

3/4 cup grapefruit juice

1 tablespoon lime juice

1/3 cup walnuts, broken

1/2 cup grapes, halved

1/2 cup red apples, diced but unpeeled

2 grapefruits, sectioned

1/4 cup apple concentrate

Dissolve gelatin in boiling water. Add grapefruit juice and lime juice. Chill until thickened. Stir in fruits, walnuts and apple concentrate. Pour into 1-1/2 quart mold and chill several hours until firm. Unmold and serve. Serves 6-8

From: "Natural Foods Cookbook" by Maxine Atwater

Tomato Salsa Salad- No Meat

1 bunch of cilantro

5-6 roma tomatoes

1 small yellow or red onion

1 small chili pepper

2 ripe avocados.

handful of whole dulse leaf

Chop cilantro, dice tomatoes, dice onion, finely dice chili pepper, dice avocado. After dicing each ingredient add to large bowl. Tear whole dulse leaf into bite size pieces, add to bowl. When finished, toss.

From: www.rawtimes.com

Salsa Fria

1 jalapeno pepper or more to taste, fresh or canned and drained, seeded and chopped fine

2 large ripe tomatoes, peeled and chopped

1 medium onion, minced

2 tablespoons olive oil

juice of 1 lemon

1/2 teaspoon dried oregano

pepper to taste

Combine all ingredients and mix well. Refrigerate covered until ready to eat.

From: "Nika Haze/ton's Way with Vegetables"

Binnie's Slaw

1/2 head of cabbage

3 or 4 carrots

1 onion

1 cup of Ray's mayonnaise (see recipe in condiments)

1 egg beaten

2 tablespoons honey

1 tablespoon fresh lemon juice

pepper to taste

Grate cabbage, carrots and onion and mix together. Make dressing by mixing beaten egg, mayonnaise, honey, lemon juice, and seasonings. Chill and serve.

From: Binnie <betten+@pitt.edu>

Fresh Mushroom Salad

2/3 cup olive oil

1/3 cup fresh lemon juice

1 teaspoon dried thyme pepper to taste

1-pound fresh mushrooms, thinly sliced

1/4 cup minced parsley

Lettuce

Combine all ingredients except the mushrooms, parsley and lettuce, and mix well. Add the mushrooms and toss with 2 forks. Cover and let stand at room temperature. At serving time, drain and sprinkle with the parsley. Pile in a serving dish lined with lettuce.

From: "Nika Haze/ton's Way with Vegetables"

Mushroom Salad

2 tablespoons fresh lemon juice

3 tablespoons olive oil

1 minced garlic clove

2 tablespoons minced fresh parsley

1 teaspoon chopped fresh oregano or 1/4 teaspoon dry

1/4 teaspoon pepper

1-pound fresh mushrooms, very thinly sliced

Combine everything but mushrooms in a medium bowl, beat with a fork to blend. Then add the mushrooms, toss to coat with dressing, and serve immediately. Delicious served with grilled meat!

From: "365 Easy Italian Recipes" by Rick Marzullo O'Connell

Black Olive Pesto

1/2 cup Black Greek or regular black olives, pitted and chopped

2 cloves of garlic, mashed, or 2 teaspoons pre-minced

1 teaspoon basil

1 shallot, quartered

1 teaspoon tarragon

2 tablespoons lemon juice

1/4 cup extra virgin olive oil

1/2 cup sundried tomatoes, oil-packed, or reconstituted in hot water for 6 minutes.

Blend all ingredients. Makes 2 cups.

From: "Cooking Healthy with One Foot out the Door"

Antipasto Chef's Salad-With Meat

Combine in a shallow dish:

1 cup chicken broth

1/2 cup olive oil

1 teaspoon marjoram

1/2 teaspoon dried oregano

1/4 teaspoon dried thyme

1/2 teaspoon honey

1/2 teaspoon pepper

dash of cayenne

1/4 cup lemon juice (substituted for red wine vinegar)

Add: 1 pound of skinless, boneless chicken breasts, poached and julienned (cut into 2 x 1/4" strips). 1/4-pound smoked ham, julienned. 1 medium red bell pepper, julienned. 1 medium green bell pepper, julienned. 1 medium onion, halved and thinly sliced. Toss to coat with marinade. Cover and marinate at room temperature for 2 hours, or refrigerate overnight, tossing occasionally. To serve, drain marinated ingredients, reserving 1/3 cup of marinade. Toss reserved marinade with: 1 head of Romaine Lettuce, rinsed, dried and torn into bite-sized pieces. Put lettuce in large salad bowls, and with a slotted spoon, arrange some of the marinated ingredients on top of each salad. Garnish with: 12 Kalamata or oil-¬cured Mediterranean olives. Serves 4 as a main dish, 6 as a first course.

Adapted from "365 Ways to Cook Chicken" by Cheryl Sedaker.

James' Salmon Salad

At my grocery store they have 2 kinds of canned salmon: one is a small (6 ounce) can, Chicken of the Sea brand, the other is generic (several brands) but all Alaskan salmon. The small can is boneless, and would no doubt be easier to eat for you. I just make a big green salad (carrots, baby greens, tomatoes, mushrooms, red/orange bell pepper, zucchini, maybe some broccoli, whatever). I add fresh crushed black pepper, some garlic powder, and some hot pepper flakes. I make a little dressing with about 2 tablespoons of orange juice and 1 tablespoon flavored olive oil (has whole herbs in the bottle). Mix all this, then just dump the salmon on top, stir it up. This tastes really great, so you should like it.

From: James Crocker <unk.gar@IX.NETCOM.COM>; Adapted by Patti Vincent

"Caveman Deli" Roast Beef Salad

This is my way to get the flavor of deli-style roast beef sandwiches without the bread. Take 1 celery stock or some other crunchy, diceable vegetable, or maybe even fruit or nuts. and dice up into 1/4" bits. Take 1 sandwich worth of roast beef (about 3 ounce depending on appetite), and chop up or pull apart into small shreds. Mix the celery (or the like) and roast beef together with a generous glob of whatever condiment or dressing you would use on the sandwich. Use enough to get a consistency similar to tuna salad. I use supermarket mayonnaise ¬horseradish sauce - the horseradish adds a great spark to it! (For purists, use Ray's mayonnaise.) Take this mixture and plop it on a bed of salad greens, or mix it into them (or, idea from Patti: Roll up in a big lettuce leaf and eat it like a burrito).

From: Kent Muller <kent@DALLAS.NET>; Adapted by Patti Vincent

SALAD DRESSINGS

Lime, Oil And Garlic Dressing

1/4 teaspoon kosher salt, plus a little more if needed

1 teaspoon finely chopped garlic

2 tablespoons finely chopped shallots

1/3 cup lime (or lemon) juice, plus extra, if needed

1 cup extra-virgin olive oil, plus extra, if needed

Freshly ground black pepper

In a small bowl, whisk the salt, garlic, and shallots with the lime juice. until the salt is dissolved. Slowly whisk in the oil until emulsified. Taste. Season with pepper and a little more salt, if needed, and add more lime juice or oil, if needed. Makes 1 1/3 cups

From: "French Food American Accent" by Debra Ponzek via Kay in RFC

Russian Salad Dressing

1 cup tomatoes (whole canned) or thick juice

1/2 cup olive oil

1/2 cup lemon juice

1 tablespoon honey

1 teaspoon paprika

1 small green onion OR

1 teaspoon onion powder

optional - 1 teaspoon horseradish powder

optional - 1 garlic clove

Blend until smooth, makes about 2 cups.

From "Ten Talents Cookbook" by Frank and Rosalie Hurd.

Tomato Dressing

1/3 cup tomato puree

1/2 cup olive oil

1/3 cup lemon juice

1 clove garlic

1 onion, chopped

1 tablespoon honey

Blend in blender until smooth.

From "Ten Talents Cookbook" by Frank and Rosalie Hurd.

Herb Dressing

Chop together very fine:

2 stalks celery and leaves

2 small green onions + tops

4 sprigs parsley

Add:

1 teaspoon paprika

1/4 teaspoon dried basil

1/8 teaspoon marjoram or rosemary

Add to above:

1 cup olive oil

2/3 cup lemon juice

Shake vigorously in tightly covered jar until well blended. Allow to stand in refrigerator until flavors are blended.

From "Ten Talents Cookbook" by Frank and Rosalie Hurd.

Salad Dressing

Olive oil and lemon juice in a three to one ratio

about 1 tablespoon of tomato paste

a couple of slices of fresh onion

approximately. 2 gloves garlic

about 2 teaspoons mustard.

Whirl in the blender and toss with hot, nuked broccoli florets. Of course, it can be used on salad.

From Beverie <abemco@COMM-PLUS.NET>

Caesar Salad Dressing Recipe

1 raw or coddled egg

3 tablespoons lemon juice

garlic

2-ounce tin anchovies with capers packed in olive oil

1 cup olive oil

Blend first three ingredients. Slowly drizzle in oil, blending continuously. Blend until dressing thickens, add anchovies, blend.

From Kathleen <Yoeschucho@AOL.COM>

CONDIMENTS

Ray's Mayonnaise

1 whole egg, at room temperature (plus 1 yolk for blender)

1/2 teaspoon dry mustard

1/4 teaspoon salt (crushed sea salt is preferable)

1/4 teaspoon white pepper (preferably fresh ground)

1 1/2 tablespoons

lemon juice

1 cup light olive oil

Combine egg, mustard, pepper, and lemon juice in blender. Cover and blend 3-5 seconds. Continue blending and slowly add olive oil in a steady even stream. Blend until mayonnaise is thick. Scrape mayo into a glass container, cover and keep refrigerated. Mayonnaise should keep one week.

From "NeanderThin: A Caveman's Guide to Nutrition"

Aioli, The Famous Garlic Mayonnaise

4-6 large garlic cloves, peeled

2 egg yolks, lightly beaten-at room temperature

about 2 cups olive oil-at room temperature

lukewarm water

juice of 1 lemon

Pound the garlic cloves to a paste. Add the egg yolks. Mix in a bowl with a wooden spoon (or use a marble mortar and wooden pestle), always turning in one direction, until the garlic and eggs have assimilated and are just beginning to get pale. While doing this, add about 4 tablespoons of oil, very very slowly, drop by drop. The mixture should be thick. Add 1 tablespoon of water and 1 teaspoon of lemon juice and continue stirring, adding the oil in a very thin stream. When the mixture gets too thick again, add 1 more teaspoon each water and lemon juice. Repeat until all oil is used. If the mayonnaise separates, Put it into a clean bowl. Add a garlic clove, 1 teaspoon of lukewarm water, and 1 egg yolk. Crush and mix together. Add the separated mayonnaise by teaspoons to the bowl, stirring constantly in one direction.

From "Nika Haze/ton's Way with Vegetables"

Lemon Mayonnaise

1 egg

pepper to taste

1 tablespoon lemon juice

3/4-1 cup olive oil

Put all ingredients into a bowl or beaker. Introduce the hand blender to base of the bowl, switch it on and hold in position until the oil emulsifies. This is also quite nice with 1/2 teaspoon of dry mustard powder and/or garlic added. For a more seafood-thousand island type dressing, simply add a tablespoonful of tomato puree.

From Braun Hand blender booklet

Ray's Catsup

3 1/2 pounds tomatoes (washed and sliced)

2 medium onions (sliced)

1/8 clove garlic

1/2 bay leaf

1/2 red pepper

1/4 cup unsweetened fruit juice (white grape, pear, or apple)

1 teaspoon whole allspice

1 teaspoon whole cloves

1 teaspoon whole mace

1 teaspoon celery seed

1 teaspoon black peppercorns

1/2-inch cinnamon stick

1/2 cup lemon juice

pinch of cayenne

pepper and salt

Boil tomatoes, onion, garlic, bay leaf, and red pepper until soft. Add fruit juice. Mix spices (allspice, cloves, mace, celery seed, peppercorns, and cinnamon) and put them into a bag. Add spice bag to mixture, boiling quickly, and stirring frequently until it reduces to half the quantity. Take out the spice bag. Add lemon juice, cayenne and salt. Continue boiling for 10 more minutes. Bottle catsup in clean jars with 3/4 inch of space above for expansion. Seal and freeze immediately. Always refrigerate container that is currently in use.

From "NeanderThin: A Caveman's Guide to Nutrition"

Cranberry Fruit Relish

1 package cranberries, washed

4-5 unpeeled apples, grated

1/4 cup raw honey, or to taste

2 small oranges (use part skin)

Run cranberries thru fine food chopper with oranges. Or process in blender until finely chopped. Combine with grated apples, add honey to taste, chill to blend flavors. Can add a few chopped pecans or grated coconut, if desired.

From: Ten Talents Cookbook by Frank and Rosalie Hurd.

Cranberry Relish For Thanksgiving

1 bag of fresh cranberries

1-2 navel oranges (Peel & removed white)

1-2 apples

nut if desired (I used pecans)

sweeten to taste (raw honey or stevia)

Chop cranberries & orange in food processor. Use as much orange as needed to keep cranberries moving so that they are finely chopped. Place in a bowl. Then chop apples in food processor. Add to cranberries Chop nuts if desired and add to cranberries. Mix well and sweeten to taste. The oranges also create the juice in the salad. So, adjust the amount of oranges based on how juicy (wet) you want your salad.

From: Patricia Cook at http://www.rawtimes.com/

CHUTNEYS

Fresh Coconut And Mint Chutney

1-2 hot jalapeno chilies, seeded and chopped

1/2-inch scrapped fresh ginger root sliced

10 whole almonds, blanched

1/3 cup water

2 tablespoons lime or lemon juice

1 tablespoon chopped dried fruit soaked in boiling water for 5-10 minutes and drained (papaya, or mango works well)

1/3 cup trimmed fresh mint, lightly packed

1 cup grated FRESH coconut, lightly packed.

Use a food processor fitted with a metal blade or a blender. With the machine running, drop in the chilies and ginger and process until minced. Add nuts, pulse four or five times until ground. Add the water, juice, dried fruit and mint, and process until smooth. Stop the machine, add the coconut, and continue to process until the chutney is creamy and smooth. To accompany dishes, it should be fairly thick as a dipping sauce it can be thinner, use coconut milk. Serve at room temperature or chilled. Makes about 1 3/4 cups, will keep covered and refrigerated for a couple of days.

From Willow <11Ji!low@VENUS.NET>

Fresh Coriander Chutney

1 teaspoon cumin seeds

3 tablespoons sesame seeds

1/4 cup FRESHLY grated coconut or 1/4 cup chopped almonds

1 cup trimmed fresh coriander, slightly packed

1-2 hot jalapenos seeded and chopped

1.2-inch scrapped fresh ginger root, chopped

2 tablespoons water

1/4 cup refrigerated coconut milk (optional)

1 tablespoon chopped dates or rehydrated raisins

Combine the cumin seeds, sesame seeds and coconuts or nuts in a heavy frying pan and place over low heat. Dry-roasting, stirring frequently, until the coconut or nuts darken a few shades. Combine the coconut mixture and the remaining ingredients in a food processor fitted with the metal blade, or a blender, and process until smooth. The texture should resemble runny apple-sauce. Transfer to a bowl and serve or cover and refrigerate. Makes 1 cup, will keep refrigerated for 2-3 days.

From Willow <11Jillow@VENUS.NET>

Creamy Almond (Or Hazelnut) Chutney

1 cup raw almonds

1/4 teaspoon lemon juice

1/2-inch piece of fresh ginger, peeled and sliced

1-2 jalapenos seeded, chopped

up to 1/3 cup of water

2 tablespoons chopped fresh coriander (cilantro)

Combine everything but the coriander in a blender or food processor, blend until smooth, adding more water if necessary to produce a loose puree. Transfer to a bowl and add the coriander, well covered, will keep for three days in refrigerator. This chutney thickens as it sits. Thin it out with water to the desired consistency.

From Willow <11Jillow@VENUS.NET>

Shredded Mango And Coconut Chutney

2 medium firm unrip mangoes

1/4 cup dried or fresh coconut ribbons

1 tablespoon diced dried fruit, such as papaya or apricot

1 tablespoon each orange and lime juice

1/8 teaspoon cayenne or paprika or a mix (depending on the heat you want)

1-2 jalapenos seeded and slivered

2 tablespoons sesame or coconut oil

1 teaspoon black mustard seeds

2 tablespoons finely chopped fresh cilantro

Peel the mangoes and coarsely shred the fruit. Discard the seed. Combine the mango with the coconut, dried fruit, juices, cayenne or paprika and green chilies in serving bowl, gently toss, cover and marinate for 1/2 hour. It can be refrigerated for up to 6 hours before serving. Heat the oil in a small pan over moderate heat until hot but not smoking. Drop in the mustard seeds and fry until they turn grey and sputter. Keep a lid handy to catch flying seeds. Pour the seeds into the salad, add the fresh coriander, toss to mix and serve.

From Willow <11Ji!low@VENUS.NET>

Pudina Ki Chatni (Mint Chutney)

2 cups fresh mint leaves

1 small onion

2 cloves garlic

1 fresh hot green chile pepper (seeded, if you prefer it milder)

1 tablespoon lemon juice

1 teaspoon cayenne pepper

3 1/2 fluid ounces water

Process all ingredients in a food processor to make a thick paste. To store, keep covered in the refrigerator. Coriander chutney can be made simply by substituting fresh coriander (cilantro) for the mint.

From: Jennifer Freeman

Peach Mint Salsa

2 ripe peaches; peeled and-diced

1 small red pepper; chopped

1/2 red onion; chopped

1 small jalapeno pepper; minced

1/4 cup pineapple juice

3 tablespoons grape juice

2 tablespoons fresh chopped mint

I created this special salsa to serve with Grilled Boneless Leg of Lamb (see recipe). Mix all ingredients together and refrigerate at least one hour to blend flavors. May be made a day or two in advance. Yields 3 cups

http://busycooks.miningco.com; Adapted by Patti Vincent

STOCKS, SAUCES & GRAVIES

Pizzaiola Sauce

1 1/2 to 2 pounds ripe tomatoes, peeled, seeded and chopped

1/4 cup olive oil

2 garlic cloves, minced

pepper, to taste

1 teaspoon dried oregano

1/4 cup minced parsley

Heat oil in a heavy pan. Add all the other ingredients. Cook over high heat, stirring all the time, for about 5 to 7 minutes, or until the tomatoes are just soft and hot. Serve with steaks.

From: Nika Haze/ton's "Way with Vegetables"

Tomato Sauce/Juice

Since many classic recipes call for tomato juice or tomato sauce, it's good to know that you can make your own rather than rely on the canned varieties that contain additives. To make tomato juice, simply puree tomatoes in a blender, add lemon juice and salt. Strain the mixture for juice and retain the pulp and a little juice to use in recipes calling for tomato juice.

From: Natural Foods Cookbook by Maxine Atwater

Basque Tomato Sauce

1/4 cup olive oil

8 cloves garlic, peeled and crushed

2 cups peeled and diced yellow onions

1 1/2 cups cored, seeded and diced green bell peppers

3 cups very ripe tomatoes, diced

1 4 ounce can whole green chiles, Mexican style, pureed

1/4 cup chopped parsley

5 cups beef stock

pepper to taste

In a 6-quart saucepan sauté the garlic, onion and green pepper in the oil until tender. Add the tomatoes, pureed chiles, and parsley and sim¬mer until very tender. Add Beef Stock. Cover and simmer 1 hour. Uncover and simmer 1 hour more to reduce and thicken the sauce. Stir occasionally, pepper to taste.

From: The Frugal Gourmet Jeff Smith

Meat Gravy

1 cup meat drippings or broth

1 cup nutmilk

1 tablespoon plus

1 teaspoon arrowroot

Add arrowroot to nutmilk and stir well. Add to dripping and cook on low stirring constantly until gravy is thickened.

From: Patti Vincent

NOTE: Arrowroot, what is it?

While the purposes are the same, there are some differences between the finished product when using arrowroot vs cornstarch. Arrowroot slurries and cornstarch slurries are both used to thicken sauces and gravies. They both yield a clear, glossy sauce which gives a "mouth feel" and appearance similar to a sauce containing quantities of butter. They both require much less time than a flour-thickened sauce. They are both used as slurries, stirred into the hot liquid *off heat! *. The arrowroot slurry is merely stirred into the liquid for 30 seconds to a minute and it's ready.

Arrowroot thickened sauces, on the other hand, freeze well in such preparations as chicken pies, and do not re-hydrolyze (the word just popped out of my sub-conscious) when the pies are reheated. I have also used it for thickening chicken ala king, which I have then frozen and re-heated without any problems.

From: p008383b@pbfreenet.seflin.lib.fl.us (Edward Conroy)

MARINADES

Cuban Lime Marinade

6 cloves garlic - minced (2 Tablespoon.)

2 teaspoons ground cumin

1 tablespoon chopped fresh oregano (or 1 teaspoon dried)

1/2 teaspoon ground black pepper

1/2 cup fresh lime juice

Place the garlic in a mortar and pestle and mash to a smooth paste (or mash in a shallow bowl with a fork). Work in the cumin, oregano, pepper, and lime juice. Add a pound of vegetables. Marinate for at least six hours, stirring occasionally. Broil or grill until done, basting occasionally with the leftover marinade. Serves 5.

Adapted from Steven Raichlen's "High-Flavor Low-Fat Cooking"

RENDERING FATS

Pork Lard

Preheat oven to 250°F. Place 1 pound of fat (leaf fat, fat back or pork fat pieces cleaned of skin and meat and finely diced) in an ovenproof dish. Add enough cold water to partially cover. Put in oven (or over very low flame) for 40 minutes, or until fat has melted, stirring occasionally to prevent it from browning or sticking. Remove from oven and strain through a cheesecloth into a heat proof container. Set aside. When fat has set into a smooth white shortening, cover and refrigerate. Will keep for 3 months.

From Amanda <ah!S@PANTHEON.com> YALE.EDU>

DRIED MEATS

Beef Jerky

For each pound of meat:

1 teaspoon salt

2 teaspoon FRESH black pepper - Fresh flavor is important!

3 teaspoon marjoram

Garlic powder - Optional

Sprinkle above ingredients onto a *THICK* steak. Pound in with mallet. Cut beef into strips and lay on oven rack with aluminum foil underneath to catch drips (If available, an arrangement like a roasting pan is perfect. Heat oven to 150°F. F and open oven door slightly to allow water to escape. Cook 7 to 8 hours, or until the meat is dry and slightly brittle - It should "splinter" when bent.

From: rec.food.cooking

Ray's Pemmican

Pemmican was relied on heavily by native North Americans when travelling. A high-energy food which keeps for an extended period of time, pemmican also makes a great snack for the urban hunter-gatherer.

1-pound suet (beef fat)

1-pound dried red meat (lean and uncooked; remove all fat before drying; 6 pounds raw lean meat yields 1-pound dried meat)

Render (melt) the suet in a pan (preferably cast iron). the suet must be rendered twice to prevent spoilage. Pound dried meat into a fine powder (a food processor will make this process much easier) and add to the twice rendered suet. While mixture is still liquid, pour into muffin pan to make pemmican cakes. If desired, wrap pemmican cakes in wax paper, as pemmican is greasy. Dried berries can be added for taste.

From "NeanderThin: A Caveman's Guide to Nutrition"

Kent's Pemmican

INGREDIENTS

* Raw red meat. Eye round roast is widely recommended. Also rump steak and London broil.

* Suet: this is a particular type of beef fat. Other types will not work correctly, so be sure you get the right stuff.

* Flavorings (optional). Salt, pepper, garlic, and dried fruit or nuts are sometimes used. One person recommended sage. If using salt, go easy on it. According to the instructions that came with my dryer, you should use at least 1 teaspoon of salt per pound of meat in order to prevent bacteria growth. You will need about 60% meat, 40% suet - these measurements are by weight, after preparation. If you have extra of either, you can save it for the next batch.

Slice and dry as you would for jerky; it must be dry enough to break rather than bend. Break it up by hand or with a food processor. Some people like it powdered, some prefer a more granular texture. Add the spices or other flavorings, if any.

"Rendering" the suet. This is the part of the process about which there is the most confusion. Apparently the idea is to remove the skins or rinds, as well as any water.

One person recommends actually adding some water at first, to prevent burning. During cooking, the water settles to the bottom and boils away. You can see the little blobs of water at the bottom of the pan; it's done when they're gone. Cut the suet into small chunks, and heat it in a pan over LOW heat - don't let it get hot enough to smoke, as it may give the pemmican a bad taste.

And have other unpleasant side effects such as adding impurities to the food, annoying your spouse, etc. The best explanation I found for this process was from Bob Baldwin. He wrote: "This process take a while and you will end up with melted fat and brown globs of stuff (it's not as gross as it sounds). Pour the whole works through a sieve into another pan (I got a large sieve at Target - it doesn't need to be giant) and discard the globs - I use a coffee can. I then put a couple of layers of cheese cloth in the sieve and filter the fat again. Now you have the fat.

Let the suet cool until it is cool enough to touch but still liquid. Pour it onto the meat slowly and mix it in until all the meat is "just saturated" (Ray) or "about the consistency of fudge" (Bob). Fill muffin tins with it, or roll it out into a sheet and cut into cookie-size chunks. When cool, it should be firm, although still a bit greasy to the touch; so, wrap it in foil, plastic, or something else that the fat won't soak through. Properly made, it should keep for years at room temperature.

From: Muller <.kent@dallas.net>

DRY RUBS

Mild Mexican Jerky

1 teaspoon salt

1/2 teaspoon crushed oregano

1/4 teaspoon pepper

1 teaspoon paprika

1 teaspoon chili powder

1/2 teaspoon garlic powder

Middle Eastern Jerky

1 teaspoon salt

1/4 teaspoon turmeric

1/8 teaspoon pepper

1/8 teaspoon ground cumin

1-1/2 teaspoons coriander

1/4 teaspoon chili powder

1/4 teaspoon ground ginger

Fiesta Jerky

1 teaspoon salt

1 teaspoon onion powder

1/4 teaspoon pepper

1/4 teaspoon ground cumin

1 tablespoon chili powder

1 teaspoon garlic powder

Curried Jerky

1 teaspoon salt

1 1/2 teaspoons curry powder

1/4 teaspoon pepper

1/2 teaspoon garlic powder

1/8 teaspoon cinnamon

1 teaspoon ground ginger

1/16 teaspoon ground cloves

1/8 teaspoon ground cumin

From: rec.food.preserving

CHILI POWDER

Firehouse Hot Chili Powder

6 tablespoons Paprika

2 tablespoons Turmeric

1 tablespoon Dried chili peppers

1 teaspoon Cumin

1 teaspoon Oregano

1/2 teaspoon Cayenne

1/2 teaspoon Garlic powder

1/2 teaspoon Salt

1/4 teaspoon Ground cloves

Mix all ingredients and grind to a fine powder using a mortar and pestle, or food processor or blender. Spice will keep 6 months or so on the pantry shelf. TO USE: This powder is somewhat more pungent and fresher tasting than a packaged brand, so use a bit less. Yields 5.5 ounce

Source: "Cheaper and Better Alternatives to Store Bought Goods," By Nancy Simes

Chili Powder

2 tablespoons Cumin seeds or 2 tablespoons ground

4 Dried hot chili peppers; ground* or 2 teaspoons crushed;

red pepper

2 teaspoons Dried oregano

2 teaspoons Garlic powder

2 teaspoons Onion powder

1 teaspoon Ground allspice

1/8 teaspoon Ground cloves

*If using dried hot chili peppers, remove the seeds before grinding or the mixture will be too hot. Combine all ingredients in a blender or electric grinder and grind until mixture is a coarse powder. recipes as directed. Yields 1/4 cup.

Source: "Rodale's Basic Natural Foods Cookbook." MM: Lyn.

HOT BEVERAGES

Chai - Tea

8 cups water

6-10 quarter sized slices of fresh ginger root

10-15 cardamom pods, cracked open

1 teaspoon of fennel seeds

4 cloves

1 or 2 pieces of dried orange rind

8-10 black peppercorns

In a sauce pan with a tight-fitting lid combine all the ingredients. Bring to a boil. Reduce heat and simmer, covered for at least 20 minutes. Simmer longer for a richer, spicier flavor. This tea can be sweetened with raw honey. You can also add almond milk or coconut milk or add one green tea bag for a stronger tea.

From: Patti Vincent

Hot Chocolate

3/4 cup pure coconut milk

1/4 cup water (If you use lite coconut milk DO NOT ADD WATER.)

1/2 tablespoon carob powder

raw honey to taste (about 1/2 tsp)

Combine coconut milk, water and carob powder. Blend with a wire whisk, heat on stove top or microwave. Add honey to taste.

From: Patti Vincent

Cranberry Tea

1-pound cranberries

1/2 cup honey

2 1/2-quart water

4 cinnamon sticks

2 teaspoons whole cloves

1 cup orange juice

In covered saucepan, combine cranberries, honey, and water; simmer until cranberries pop; add cinnamon sticks and cloves; continue to simmer until it smells good. Add orange juice. Strain and keep juice (use pulp in other recipes). 1 tablespoon lemon juice can be added to tea, if desired. Serve warm.

From: Donna (in CA) <1adibugz77@aol.com>. posted in RFC; Adapted by Patti Vincent

Holiday Wassail

1 can (16 ounces) apricot halves, undrained

4 cups unsweetened pineapple juice

2 cups apple cider

1 cup orange juice

18 whole cloves

6 cinnamon sticks (3-1/2 inches), broken

Additional cinnamon sticks, optional

Apricots lend golden color and goodness to this fruity beverage

In a blender or food processor, blend apricots and liquid until smooth. Pour into a large saucepan. Add pineapple juice, cider and orange juice. Place the cloves and cinnamon sticks in a double thickness of cheesecloth; bring up corners of cloth and tie with a string to form a bag. Add to saucepan. (Or place loose spices in saucepan and strain before serving.) Bring to a boil. Reduce heat; cover and simmer 15-20 minutes. Serve hot in mugs. Garnish with cinnamon sticks if desired. Yields 2 quarts.

From: http://cyou.com!-christmas!recipes!beverage.htm

COLD BEVERAGES

Cantaloupe Smoothie

I just take half a cantaloupe, clean and peel it, and slice it up into chunks. Then put it in a blender, with 4-6 ice cubes and enough water to cover the cantaloupe. (If you have a small blender, you can use smaller amounts of everything.) Then blend it on HIGH for about a minute. When it's whipped up, it has a sweet, creamy consistency, which is perfect for anybody who craves drinking milk. I don't, but I love this smoothie.

From: Shawn <75537.1154@compuserve.com>

Fresh Coconut Milk

I decided to be a bit adventurous on this one. Having read on the can that coconut milk is made from steamed coconut, I figured I could make it fresh. I bought a coconut and after much effort, and several friends making suggestions, I finally got it open. Actually, a hammer and screwdriver work best. Then I took the meat out and boiled it with bottled water. One medium coconut made about 6 cups of milk/broth. I imagine it will work the same. You can then put the milk & some ice in a blender and made a frosty coconut shake.

From: Gaylen <mtharp2668@aol.com>

Home-Made Strawberry Lemonade

8 cups water

1 cup fresh-cut strawberries

1 cup frozen strawberries

honey to taste

1 cup lemon juice

2 lemons sliced

In a large container, combine 4 cups of water and the fresh and frozen strawberries. Let soak in the sun for 3-4 hours. In another container, combine the lemon juice, sliced lemons and water. Chill for 3-4 hours to let the lemon juice soak thru. Mix the 2 containers together, and add honey to your taste. Serve chilled over ice.

From: "Cooking with the Dead" by Elizabeth Zipem

NUT MILKS

Note: For Nut and Seed Milks Using the same equipment, ratio of ingredients, and procedure, you can make wonderful milks from sesame seeds, sunflower seeds, or cashews.

You need:

a simple blender or Vita-Mix

one medium-size fine strainer

cheesecloth to line the strainer (optional)

a large bowl

a pitcher with lid, for storage

Almond Milk

1/2 cup shelled raw almonds

1/2 tablespoon pure maple syrup (optional) or small amount of Stevia.(ed.)

2 cups water

Blanch almonds by placing them in 1 cup boiling water. Allow them to stand until the water has cooled slightly, and then peel off skins, or prepare milk with unblanched almonds. (Milk from blanched almonds will be slightly whiter in color and smoother in consistency with no difference in flavor.) Dry almonds well.

1. Place almonds in blender and grind to a fine powder. Add sweetener and 1 cup water. Blend again for 1 to 2 minutes to form a smooth cream.

2. With blender running on high, add remaining cup of water slowly through opening of blender lid. Blend 2 minutes.

3. Place the strainer over a large bowl; to ensure a smooth milk, line the strainer with cheesecloth. (If you do not have cheesecloth, you can simply strain your milk twice, using an even finer strainer the second time.)

4. Pour almond milk slowly into strainer and allow to filter through. Add liquid to strainer in increments and just let it drain naturally, or stir the milk in the strainer with a spoon to encourage it to pass through more rapidly.

5. When all the milk has passed through the strainer, there will be approximately 1/2 cup of almond fiber accumulated. If you have used a cheesecloth liner, you can pull the edges together and gently squeeze the remaining milk out of the fiber, or use a spoon to gently press the remaining milk through the strainer. (The fiber can be stored in the refrigerator for a few days and used as a moisturizing body scrub when you shower.) Makes about 2 cups. Note: The amount can be doubled if you need a quart of Almond Milk. Almond Milk will keep in the refrigerator for 4 or 5 days. Store it in a jar or pitcher with an airtight lid.

From: "The American Vegetarian Cookbook" by Marilyn Diamond. Via: Cathy Flick on Yeast-l list

SPECIAL OCCASIONS

Hors D'oeuvres

Fresh Cilantro Salsa

2 cloves garlic

1 large onion, quartered

1 green bell pepper, quartered & seeded

3 to 4 jalapeno peppers

6 tomatoes, peeled, seeded and chopped or 2 cans (16 ounce each) plum tomatoes, drained and chopped

1 cup fresh cilantro

some salt to taste

freshly ground pepper to taste

1. place the garlic in the bowl of a food processor and process until it is minced. Add the onion and peppers and process with on/off pulses until they are barely chopped.

2. Add the tomatoes and cilantro and process until combined but slightly chunky. Add salt and pepper. Refrigerate until ready to use. Yields 2 & 1/2 cups.

From: "Charleston Receipts"

Crudities

There are always many things available in the markets that can be used for this:

asparagus (very young only)

broccoli

carrots

cauliflower

celery

cherry tomatoes

mushrooms

peppers: yellow, red, green

radishes

scallions

squashes: zucchini, pale green, yellow

sugar snap peas (not paleo, for guests)

Mushroom And Shrimp Antipasto

1 celery rib, halved

1/2 small onion

1 sprig fresh thyme or 1 teaspoon dried

1/2 lemon plus 1 tablespoon fresh lemon juice

3 whole peppercorns, crushed

1/8 teaspoon hot pepper flakes

1/2 cup chopped tomato

1/8 teaspoon pepper

8 ounces fresh mushrooms, quartered

12 romaine lettuce leaves

12 ounces medium shrimp, shelled and de-veined

1/2 cup mayonnaise (use a DE compliant recipe)

1 tablespoon chopped fresh basil or 1/2 teaspoon dried

In a nonreactive saucepan, bring the 6 cups of water to a boil, with the celery, thyme, 1/2 lemon, peppercorns and hot pepper flakes. Boil 3 minutes. Plunge shrimp into boiling water and cook until they just turn pink, 2-3 minutes. Drain in a colander and rinse under cold running water. Transfer shrimp to a bowl; discard vegetables and lemon half. In a small bowl, combine mayo, tomato, basil, pepper and 1 tablespoon lemon juice. Beat with a fork to blend. Add mushrooms and shrimp and toss to coat. Pile salad onto lettuce leaves.

Prom: "365 Easy Italian Recipes" by Rick Marzullo O'Connell

Shrimp Cocktail

1-pound shrimp

6 tablespoons chili sauce

2 tablespoons lemon juice

1/2 tablespoon horseradish

1/4 teaspoon grated onion

1/3 cup finely chopped celery

Crisp salad greens (2 cups leaves)

lemon wedges

Cook and clean shrimp. cover and chill. Combine chili sauce, lemon juice, horseradish, onion to make cocktail sauce. Stir. Mix chilled shrimp with celery. Line cocktail cups with salad greens. Spoon in shrimp mixture. Spoon on some sauce. Garnish with lemon wedges.

Prom: Pam at http://www.ilovejesus.comllotllocarbl

Cold Shrimp Stuffed Avocados

3 large avocados

juice of 1 lemon

1-pound cooked shelled shrimp (reserve 6 whole shrimp), coarsely chopped

1 hot chili pepper, peeled if fresh, seeded, washed and chopped fine

1 hard-cooked egg, chopped

2 dozen pitted green or black olives, chopped

mayonnaise

pepper

3 tablespoons minced fresh coriander leaves or parsley

Cut avocados in half lengthwise, pit, and scoop out the flesh. Put the flesh into a bowl, then sprinkle the shells with a little lemon juice to prevent darkening. Mash the avocado flesh with a fork. Add the shrimp, hot pepper, egg and olives and mix well. Add enough mayonnaise, beginning with 1/3 cup, to bind the ingredients together. Pepper to taste. Stuff the avocado shells with this mixture. Top each with one of the reserved shrimp and sprinkle with coriander. 6 servings.

Prom: "Nika Haze/ton's Way with Vegetables"

FRUITS

Apple Peach Walnuts Cream

1 apple

2 peaches or nectarines

1 cup walnuts (soaked overnight)

4-5 dates (fresh or dried)

For all mixtures: blend the ingredients in a blender for few seconds

From: www.rawtimes.com

Apricot Yummies

Sun-dried unsulfured apricots

Raw walnuts

Mix together equal parts of ground apricots and walnuts (Run through coarse food grinder). Shape into flat squares or balls. May be rolled in shredded coconut. These freeze very well.

From: "Ten Talents Cookbook" by Frank and Rosalie Hurd.

Fruity Chews

Put thru a food grinder:

1 cup dates

1 cup dried apricots, unsulfured

1 cup raisins

1 cup walnuts or pecans

Add in and mix:

1 cup coconut shreds

3 tablespoons fresh lemon juice

Pack smooth into flat pan lined with waxed paper. Chill and cut into squares. May be rolled in fine coconut. Can be made into balls and flattened with a walnut half. Freeze well.

From: "Ten Talents Cookbook" by Frank and Rosalie Hurd.

Cinnamon Apple Chips

2 cups unsweetened apple juice

1 cinnamon stick

2 Red Delicious apples

In large skillet or pot, combine apple juice and cinnamon stick; bring to a low boil while preparing apples. With sharp knife, slice off 1/2 inch from top and bottom of apples and discard (or eat!). Stand apples on either cut end and gently slice crosswise into very thin (1/8 inch) rings, rotating the apple as necessary to get even slices. Drop apple slices into boiling juice; cook 4 to 5 minutes until apple slices appear translucent and lightly golden. Meanwhile, heat oven to 250°F. With slotted spatula, remove apple slices from juice and pat dry. Arrange slices on cake-cooling racks, being sure none overlap. With pot holder (rack will become hot from chips) place racks on middle shelf in oven; bake 30 to 40 minutes until apple slices are lightly browned and almost dry to touch. Let chips completely cool on racks before storing in air ¬tight container. Makes 2 servings.

From: Clelia <cmd@ICA.NET>

Peach Butter

Peaches (at least 8-12)

Optional raw honey or pure maple syrup (was sugar)

Lemon juice, if desired

Spices, if desired

Peel and pit the peaches. Quarter them. Put the quartered peaches in a heavy kettle and add about 1-2 cups of water to the pot. Start cook¬ing over low heat to discourage sticking. Cook until tender, stirring often to discourage sticking. After cooking, drain the peaches through a colander, reserving juice (you can make jelly with the resultant juice). Put the peaches through a food mill to puree. A blender or food processor can be used, though their action is different than milling. I much prefer a food mill - it strains to puree and separates any extraneous fiber; then blender chop to puree. The final texture is different. Measure the pulp/puree by volume. Put it into a heavy bottom kettle. Add some sweetener if you wish. Add a wee splash of lemon juice at this point, if you wish. Commence cooking over low to moderate heat, uncovered, stirring to dissolve the sugar. Don't sit down and read the paper. Don't leave the room. When the stuff begins to boil, reduce the heat to very low, put a splatter screen atop and cook until it is thickened to your liking. If you want spiced butter, add spices towards the end of the cooking. I won't give amounts of spices: Start with a small amount. Be careful with ground cloves-a little goes a long way. Spices that are nice with peach butter include cinna¬mon and nutmeg.

If you leave the room to get on with your life, take a timer with you and set it for 5-10 minutes (your cue to run back and stir and check) - less time as it gets closer to being done. When you've got the stuff cooking, go back to that reserved juice and strain it, hot, through about 3-4 layers of cheesecloth. Use the juice for peach jelly (check a pectin box for a recipe) or adding it to bar-becue sauce.

Fruit butters are great! They are very interruptible. If you are uncertain as to whether or not they are done, hold everything! Get the pot off the heat and let it and the contents cool. Check the texture and consistency then. If it's as you like it, reheat and jar. I've taken three days to make my apricot butter if I haven't had the necessary time to do it in one shot. Expect the volume to have reduced by about one-third. Use that guide for determining how many canning jars to prepare. Have your canning jars and lids prepared and ready to fill.

When the butter is thickened, fill the jars, remove bubbles, seal and process in a boiling water bath for 10 minutes. Because of the density of fruit butter, I like to have my batch bubbling hot when I fill my jars. I do this by returning the now done butter to my mixing pitcher and nuking it till the edges are bubbling. Then I pour it into the jars, check for bubbles and seal and process.

I recognize that this might be seen as a pretty involved process. It's worth the time.

Other Fruit Butters

Same method.

Apricot Butter - I don't like mine spiced at all! *Maybe* a wee splash of orange juice, more likely not. Do what you will. Easy on the lemon juice if you use it.

Plum Butter - My plums, when pureed, are sour and strong. They can stand cinnamon, clove, and freshly ground allspice. Skip the lemon juice.

Apple Butter - There are a zillion recipes for apple butter. Most include cinnamon, cloves, nutmeg, maybe mace. Skip the lemon juice.

Most fruit butters, because of their tanginess and spiciness are very nice with grilled or roast meats, pork and chicken in particular.

Apricot butter is a nice dip for chicken when it's cut with some lemon juice. Plum butter, too.

Adapted from: Schaller"Barb@htc.honeywell.com via rec.food.preserving

FROZEN DESSERTS

Apple Ice Kreme

This light and refreshing dessert takes a simple apple and makes you feel like you are eating something positively sinful. Use sweet apples. If you use a tart apple, like Granny Smith, you may find that you need to use a lot more maple syrup than the recipe calls for to achieve the level of sweetness most people like in a dessert.

2 cups applesauce (made by putting several peeled and cored apples through the Champion with blank)

2 cups apple juice

2 tablespoons pure maple syrup

2 teaspoons lemon juice

Puree in blender or food processor. Place in shallow dish and freeze. Serve by scraping into curls with a soup spoon or ice cream scoop. Variation: Add a scoop or two of Apple Ice Kream to chilled Sparkling apple cider or apple juice for a special drink.

Note: try this with peaches, strawberries, raspberries, blueberries, kiwi, oranges, tangerines, etc.

From: Nomi Shannon, http://www.living-foods.com!rawgoumiet

Frozen Banana Dessert

1 banana almond, hazelnut or sunflower butter (Walnut Acres) shredded fresh coconut. Spread nut butter on outside of banana, roll in coconut and freeze.

From: Binnie <betten+@pitt.edu>

Frozen Fruit Treat Birthday Cake

1 Bunt Cake Pan

16 ounce of dried organic figs, soaked overnight in distilled water*

16 ounce of dried pitted organic dates, soaked overnight in distilled water*

12-ounce bag of organic almonds

2 big bunches fully ripe bananas (organic if possible)

Soak fruit in separate bowls. The water level for soaking is about half full. Do not cover the dried fruits completely. Remove stems from soaked figs, puree figs and set aside. Puree dates put in sep¬arate bowl, chop almonds in food processor or blender and set aside in its own container.

Peel and puree the bananas in a blender or food processor.

To Build the Cake: Place almonds in the bottom of the mold; 2nd layer, pureed figs; 3rd layer almonds; 4th layer pureed bananas, almonds, dates, almond, figs or whatever order you desire. Almonds should be the first layer and end with dates or figs the last layer. Cover and freeze overnight.

To Serve: Remove from the freezer, place upside down on a plate and allow to sit a few minutes until thawed enough to release from the pan. Can be carefully set in warm water just long enough to release the cake, being very careful not to get water in the cake. This cake has so many possibilities. Use strawberries and blueberries for a beautiful, healthy 4th of July cake. Any of your favorite fruits can be used to make a new family tradition!

From Gracie Gordon, http://www.hacres.com

Hans' Summer "Ice Cream"

Now you don't have to be jealous on friends cooling down with some ice cream in the summer heat any more. Just take some berries out of your freezer (or the supermarket freezer) put in the food processor/blender and grind until you have something like berry-snow. Then put in one (or more) fresh egg, and blend again until thoroughly mixed. You will have to find the desired proportions yourself; it depends on the kind of berries. Do not let the berries thaw too much. I have got the best results so far with lingons. Strawberries I cut in smaller pieces before putting in the blender. If you want it sweeter, add a little honey with the egg.

From: Hans Kypounderg <lwns-k@ALGONET.SE>

Watermelon Freeze

4 cups seeded and cubed watermelon

2 cups cubed cantaloupe

3 fresh mint leaves or 1 mint tea bag

1 cup water

juice of 1 fresh lemon

Puree the melons in a food processor until smooth. Place in a saucepan and simmer 15 minutes. Meanwhile, in another pan, simmer the mint leaves or tea bag in the water about 3 minutes. Strain and add this infusion to the cooked melons. Turn off the heat and stir in the lemon juice. Line a muffin pan with cupcake liners [Note: DE followers might not have muffin pans or cupcake liners - borrow from your neighbors. Or else just use Dixie cups]. Pour the melon puree into each one and freeze. When beginning to firm up, you may insert flat wooden sticks into each treat. Freeze until completely hard or the papers will not peel easily away. Remove papers before serving. Makes 12-18.

From: "Cooking the Whole Foods Way" by Christina Pire/lo.

DESSERT SAUCES

Whipped Coconut Cream

I've discovered how to make delicious whipped cream to top on berries and fruits really easy to make. Just take a can of unsweetened coconut milk (Thai is a great brand), pour it into a jar and shake vigorously. Let sit in the refrigerator and you have a very stiffly beaten cream. Drizzle a little honey on top for sweetness if desired when you scoop it onto your dessert.

From: Ella <ellalane@AOL.COM>

One could add fruit and or spices to the coconut milk for a different flavor. Or maybe something like the spiced nuts chopped and sprinkled as a topping.

From: Patti Vincent

CANDY AND CONFECTIONS

Almond Stuffed Dates

A "sugary" treat that seems Diet Evolution enough is gooey dates, each with a roasted almond shoved inside. We did this over Christmas, and I ate these (mostly) instead of tempting cookies and things. We used raw, unsalted whole almonds, and roasted them ourselves.

Roast them on medium-high heat dry, right in a frying pan. Just sit there and watch them carefully to make sure they don't burn, moving them around and stuff. Then cool, and shove one each inside a date. I like the gooiest dates for this. Very tasty, and not too caloric if you only eat a few!

BTW- these are good for potassium and fiber, and trace minerals like calcium, zinc , etc.

Also, the oven would work just fine. I might use the broiler in this case, but still watch them very carefully. When done, they might have a hint of black on the spot where they touched the metal.

From: James Crocker

Spicy Pecans

1/4 cup raw honey

4 teaspoons cinnamon

1 1/2 teaspoons ginger

3/4 teaspoon nutmeg

1/2 teaspoon ground cloves

1/2 teaspoon ground cayenne

2 egg whites

5 cups pecan halves (or walnuts)

In small bowl, combine sugar, cinnamon, ginger, nutmeg, cloves and cayenne. In large bowl, whisk egg whites until frothy: add honey, whisk again just until egg whites and honey are combined. Add nuts a cup at a time in the egg and honey mixture. Remove and toss in the spices. Repeat again until all the nuts have been coated. Spread on 2 lightly greased baking sheets; bake at 250 for one-hour, rotating sheets halfway through baking, or until coating is crisp and nuts are fragrant. Let cool.

From: December 1995 issue of Canadian living Magazine Adapted by Patti Vincent

BREAD, PANCAKES, MUFFINS, AND COOKIES

Mock Walnut Bread

1 cup walnuts

1 egg

sea salt

Chop up the walnuts as fine as possible in a food processor then added one whole egg. The dough will be a bit sticky. Lightly coated a small cast iron pan with side pork grease (not much). Press some of the dough into a flat round and cook it turning once. Salt to taste. If you have ever made tortillas using masa flour, this is kind of the same thing only with Diet Evolution ingredients. It could be used for open faced sandwiches.

From: Patti Vincent

De Correct Pancakes

1 egg

1/4 cup of ground almonds

1/4 cup of coconut milk

Cook as regular pancakes in coconut butter or other fat. Sometimes I cook this as I would an oven pancake: Preheat oven. Heat the pan (a cast iron frying pan works the best) in a 425°F. oven until hot, add some olive oil, coconut butter, or coconut oil to the pan (1 Tablespoon) and then add the egg mixture. Cook for 10 minutes. No turning. It won't puff up like the ones made with rice flour instead of almonds, but it tastes good. There are many recipes for Puffed or Oven pancake on a Search, but almonds make it DE compliant and in my opinion tastier! It resembles Yorkshire Pudding, but with almonds it doesn't puff up very well. The pancake simply slides out of the pan because of all the grease, so it shouldn't break apart.

From: Susan Carmack

Almond Muffins

1 cup almond butter

1 cup sliced raw almonds

1 cup pure coconut milk

2 cups shredded unsweetened coconut

3 eggs

Beat and pour in muffin cups. Cook at 400°F. for 15 minutes.

From Kathleen <Yoeschucho@AOL.COM>

Cookie And Pie Crust Recipe

2 cups walnuts

1/8 cup raw, unfiltered honey (more or less to taste)

1 tablespoon cinnamon

2 egg whites (whisked until frothy)

Grind nuts and cinnamon in blender or food processor. Stir in honey. Combine with egg whites.

Drop by teaspoon on oiled cookie sheet. Bake at 350°F. for 15 minutes. Cookies will be soft; do not overbake. Makes 15 cookies. I think this would work well for a pie crust too.

Adapted from USA Weekend by Patti Vincent.

"Cookies"

1 cup almond butter

1 whole egg or white (if using whole, use medium or smaller)

2 tablespoons unsweetened applesauce

1/2 cup of raisins (or other chopped dried fruit)

2-3 tablespoons desiccated unsweetened coconut

Beat all ingredients together. It should be thick batter, but not as thick as cookie dough. Drop by tablespoons on a cookie sheet. Bake in oven (around 375°F.) until they start to go golden, about 10-12 minutes. Allow to cool, then eat! Sometimes I add a couple of teaspoons of honey or fruit juice sweetened jelly, or some dried orange peel, cinnamon or allspice, whatever I'm in the mood for.

From Amanda <ah/5@PANTHEON YALE.EDU>

STUFFING

De Correct Poultry Stuffing

2 cups finely ground blanched almonds

1 cup chopped onion (use chopped dried onion for a better flavor)

1/2 cup chopped celery (optional)

1 teaspoon ground sage

1 teaspoon ground thyme

chopped parsley

1 tablespoon mild-flavored oil (more if it seems too dry)

pepper to taste

Mix together all ingredients. Fill cavity of bird with the mixture, then roast.

From: Cecilia Thornton-Egan <ieos@surmetcity.com.au>

Sausage And Mushroom Dressing

4 onions, thinly sliced

2 to 4 tablespoons olive oil

4 cups of mushrooms (regular white or oyster mushrooms will do)

pepper

1/2 cup chicken broth

2 tablespoons side pork grease

2 pounds turkey sausage

tarragon (or maybe sage)

Sauté the onions in olive oil over medium/low heat until caramelized for about 30 minutes. Turn up the heat and add the mushrooms. Sauté them until crisp around edges about 10-15 minutes. Season with pepper. Turn the heat on high and add wine (or chicken broth) If you using wine let it cook off, if you use chicken broth just add it and let simmer.

Let this simmer mushrooms and all for about 10 minutes. Then add the grease. 1 tablespoon at a time until combined. Remove from heat and set aside. Then brown the sausage. After it's cooked thoroughly add to the mushroom mixture along with the tarragon or sage and combine thoroughly. Then either stuff it in your turkey or bake like regular dressing.

From: msmystic@aol.com on the Atkins mailing list

ABOUT THE AUTHOR

Charles Hunt

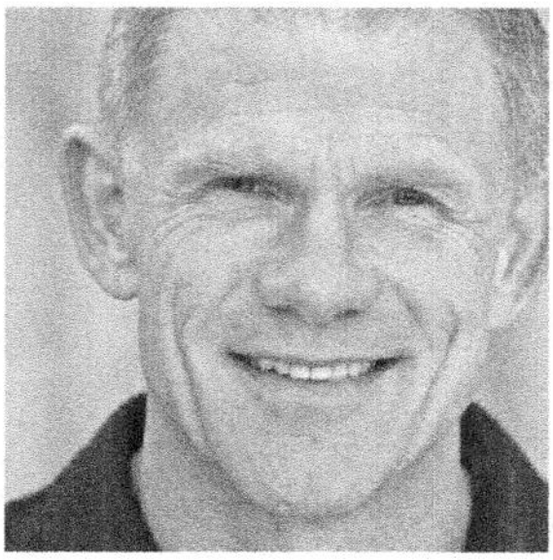

CJ Hunt, filmmaker and broadcast journalist, is the writer, co-executive producer and on camera host of January 2013's #1 Top-Selling Documentary and #1 Top-Selling Independent Film on iTunes, in both the USA and Canada.

This book, and his investigative documentary "The Perfect Human Diet", evolved from his true-life story, beginning in 1978 when paramedics brought Mr. Hunt back to life at the age of 24 after suffering a full cardiac arrest while jogging.

That incident evoked an intense passion to find out how we can all achieve longer, healthier and happier lives and then share that information with others.

With over twenty years in broadcasting, voiceovers, television and live events, Mr. Hunt currently lives in Southern California, and is the author of three books on diet and health.

RESOURCES

Books

The Paleo Thyroid Solution
by Elle Russ
www.elleruss.com

Protein Power
by Michael R. Eades, M. D. and Mary Dan Eades, M.D.
www.proteinpower.com

Protein Power LifePlan
by Michael R. Eades, M. D. and Mary Dan Eades, M.D.
www.proteinpower.com

NeanderThin: Eat Like a Caveman to Achieve a Lean, Strong, Healthy Body
by Raymond V. Audette with Troy Gilchrist
www.NeanderThin.com

Dr. Bernstein's Diabetes Solution
by Dr. Richard K. Bernstein, M.D.
www.diabetes-book.com

Websites

"The Paleolithic Diet Page" (everything you could ask for and more)
by Don Wiss
www.PaleoDiet.com

"The Paleolithic Eating Support List's Recipe Collection"
by Don Wiss
www.PaleoFood.com

BOOKS BY THIS AUTHOR

The Perfect Human Diet

The Perfect Human Diet, the companion book to the number one film, is a game changer in the world of health and nutrition. The result of broadcast journalist C.J. Hunt's unprecedented global exploration for a solution to our exploding epidemic of obesity and diet-related disease– the #1 killer in America. It's a fascinating treasure hunt - the unexpected discovery of the authentic human diet - and The Perfect Human Diet's doctor proven solution for achieving optimal human health and longevity.

Fascinating and compelling, you get the secrets about the perfect human diet that were previously unknowable - no more dietary theories from diet guru's to misguide you - The Perfect Human Diet gives you the facts. Uniquely easy to put into use, C.J. explains a new method of eating to optimize your health based on these breakthrough scientific facts, including detailed grocery shopping advice and great tasting recipes.

Described as "irrefutable" and "the answer to the obesity epidemic," The Perfect Human Diet will forever change the way you think about food, and guide you to the health and life you deserve.

Made in the USA
Monee, IL
04 November 2026

67380482R00144